HARDCORE
bodybuilding

THE BLOOD, SWEAT AND TEARS OF PUMPING IRON

---

by *Robert Kennedy*
editor of MuscleMag International

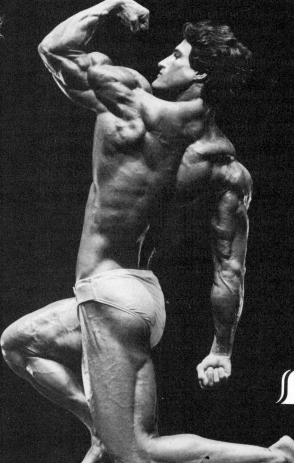

Sterling Publishing Co., Inc. New York

Dedication

To my parents,
Doris and William,
for everything

THE WOMEN'S EXERCISES

Model: Laura Davies, Canadian women's champion.
Photographs: Chris Lund
Equipment: Courtesy of Sports and Fitness Academy, Stoney Creek,
Ontario.

Library of Congress Cataloging in Publication Data

Kennedy, Robert, 1938–
  Hardcore bodybuilding.

  Includes index.
  1. Bodybuilding. I. Title. II. Title: Hard core
body building. III. Title: Hard core bodybuilding.
GV546.5.K45   1982   646.7′5   82-50549
ISBN 0-8069-4166-9
ISBN 0-8069-4167-7 (lib. bdg.)
ISBN 0-8069-7646-2 (pbk.)

  23 25 27 29 30 28 26 24 22

Copyright © 1982 by Robert Kennedy
Published by Sterling Publishing Co., Inc.
387 Park Avenue South, New York, N.Y. 10016
Distributed in Canada by Sterling Publishing
% Canadian Manda Group, P.O. Box 920, Station U
Toronto, Ontario, Canada M8Z 5P9
Distributed in Great Britain and Europe by Cassell PLC
Artillery House, Artillery Row, London SW1P 1RT, England
Distributed in Australia by Capricorn Ltd.
P.O. Box 665, Lane Cove, NSW 2066
Manufactured in the United States of America
All rights reserved

Contents

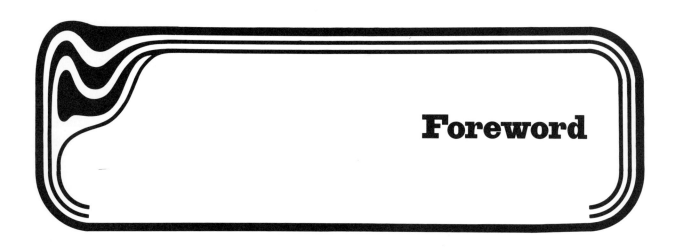

Foreword

Your chest is feeling thicker, larger. The pecs are heavier . . . the pump is not far away. You sit on the end of the exercise bench, and as you roll your body backwards to lie face up, your head barely misses the loaded barbell. You have done it a thousand times before: the surroundings, the bench, the bar are familiar.

You stare up at the heavy iron little more than a foot above your face, shuffle your feet and jiggle your "glutes" so that your entire body is balanced solidly, ready to launch the bar into space if necessary. Both hands grab the knurling instinctively, leaving equal distance from either collar. You check visually and move one hand out a tenth of an inch. HUPP! The bar rises, bearing down hard against the thumbless palms of your hands. To the uninitiated it appears precariously balanced, but you know better. You gulp air and your waist vanishes into your chest, now swelling and surging with newly summoned strength. The bar lowers slowly to your sternum, kissing the pecs with light precision, which in turn signals the triceps and pectorals to propel the weight upwards. As they straighten, you explode air from your lungs like a noisy piston and once again throw your muscles into reverse. The bar lowers to the sternum. Smoothly, cautiously, the weight rises . . . falls . . . rises. Only at the tenth repetition does invigoration and confidence yield to stress and anxiety. You counter by mentally reasserting your aggressiveness. A curse forms on your lips. The bar

has to go up two more times. Sweat stings your eyes. You blink repeatedly to focus on the bar which shakes from the diminishing control at the end of your extended arms. Momentarily you question attempting the painful madness of two more reps. Your muscles read your mind's doubt and the bar feels even heavier. It drops a fraction and your shaking arms feel limp. Give in to fatigue? The question lurks for a long second. . . .

As concentration returns, so does determination. It *will* be two more reps. You summon the needed force by huffing and puffing out air and spittle. Your grip tightens on the knurled chrome. You lower the bar. The kiss becomes a solid thump and your glutes rise slightly. Halfway up, the bar falters and the center of your chest explodes into spasms of searing hot needles. Your eyes zero in on the bar as your hearing deserts you and the weight inches up to arm's length. You've crashed through the pain barrier with *one* more rep to go.

With legs twitching, kicking out to alleviate the pent-up electricity, you take three quick gasps for oxygen to see you through the last five seconds of agony. A whispered word from your training partner, "One more!", spirits through your mind to give you extra courage. Ominously the bar comes down for the final exertion, almost out of control. As it rams into your chest and bounces into orbit, a fleeting thought of failure strikes again, but is instantly killed in a burst of iron determination to finish the job . . .

and the bar continues to climb. Your face catches fire, veins swell, temples pound, and with teeth-clenched courage, amid hellish pain shooting through your pectorals, you "growl" the weight skyward. As the arms straighten and elbows lock, the weight falls away into the welcome hands of a training partner; you stomp your feet rapidly on the floor to chase the pain from your body. It slides away and you curl up from the bench—the beastly "burn" has turned to wondrous warmth. The set is over. The "pump" has arrived!

The beauty of bodybuilding is that you can change your appearance. By your own efforts you can add or subtract pounds of body weight. You can build your arms, shoulders, legs, chest, back, and in so doing, you can get a pleasure from training you might never have dreamed possible. Even the pain has its reward: It is invariably followed by the most desirable effect of all—the pump.

This book accompanies you through the motions you know so well already. In text and photographs, the world's most advanced hardcore bodybuilding techniques are discussed and dissected. I hope it will inspire you to go the extra distance to greatness.

Use this book to break out with new enthusiasm for your bodybuilding workouts and take yourself to higher plateaus of physical perfection. Greater success *can* be yours. Here are all the advanced techniques and principles to "force-feed" your muscles to titanic new dimensions.

You will always hear differing views on bodybuilding: Do's and don'ts that seem to contradict eath other, eating suggestions that appear to conflict and exercise techniques that seem at odds. Don't worry about it.

Your body's growth depends on change. You have to surprise your muscles now and again, confuse them, pound them out. Progression is the whole point. Vary the intensity, the angle of approach, the workout length, the sets and reps—but always go for more, more, more. Don't, however, suddenly shift exercises, i.e., jump from, say, performing heavy squats right into vigorous thigh extensions without first warming up each area with light weights gradually. That can only lead to muscle tear.

This book contains the collective wisdom of the pros: sound advice, tumultuous techniques, flamboyant ideas, all designed to help you crash through your present sticking point. But nothing will happen unless you make it. Your development will reflect your total effort. Bring intensity, enthusiasm, regularity and courage to your training and you cannot possibly fail.

Accept the challenge to go all the way to bodybuilding stardom. Why not? You're young now. Life is fleetingly short. Make tonight's workout different from all previous ones. Make it your first step to real physical greatness. Is it trite to remind you that we live but once? This minute I want you to decide that you will push your limits, surpass your present point of development, venture on, on to that privileged spot at the top of the ladder—reserved one future day exclusively for you!

Appreciation

A book is not just the brainchild of one author. I owe a vote of thanks to many people:

First, to the bodybuilders themselves who appear within these pages. They are a great lot: Egos rise and fall, differences come and go, but it takes guts and determination to keep pumping iron, and that is the bond that unites us all. I respect each champion for bringing something unique to the sport.

To Pete Grymkowski and Tim Kimber of Gold's Gym and Joe Gold of World Gym, who run the two greatest hardcore bodybuilding establishments on earth, I extend heartfelt gratitude for your kindnesses. Other gyms that were very helpful include Mr. Fitness (Toronto), Bilotta's (Vancouver) and Vic Tanny's Super Fitness (Toronto).

Also, to International Federation of Body Builders (IFBB) head Ben Weider whose open house policy keeps American bodybuilding healthy and vibrant, my respect and thanks.

I offer my appreciation to photographers Garry Bartlett, an indomitable Canadian who always keeps me in high spirits, Denie from New York City, who not only took photographs for this book, but also offered numerous ideas for which I am especially grateful, and to Al Antuck, Doris Barrilleaux, Bill Reynolds and the enigmatic Britisher Chris Lund, who made special trips to California to capture the reality of bodybuilding with his magic lens. Most of this book's photographs are proof of his acute artistic eye.

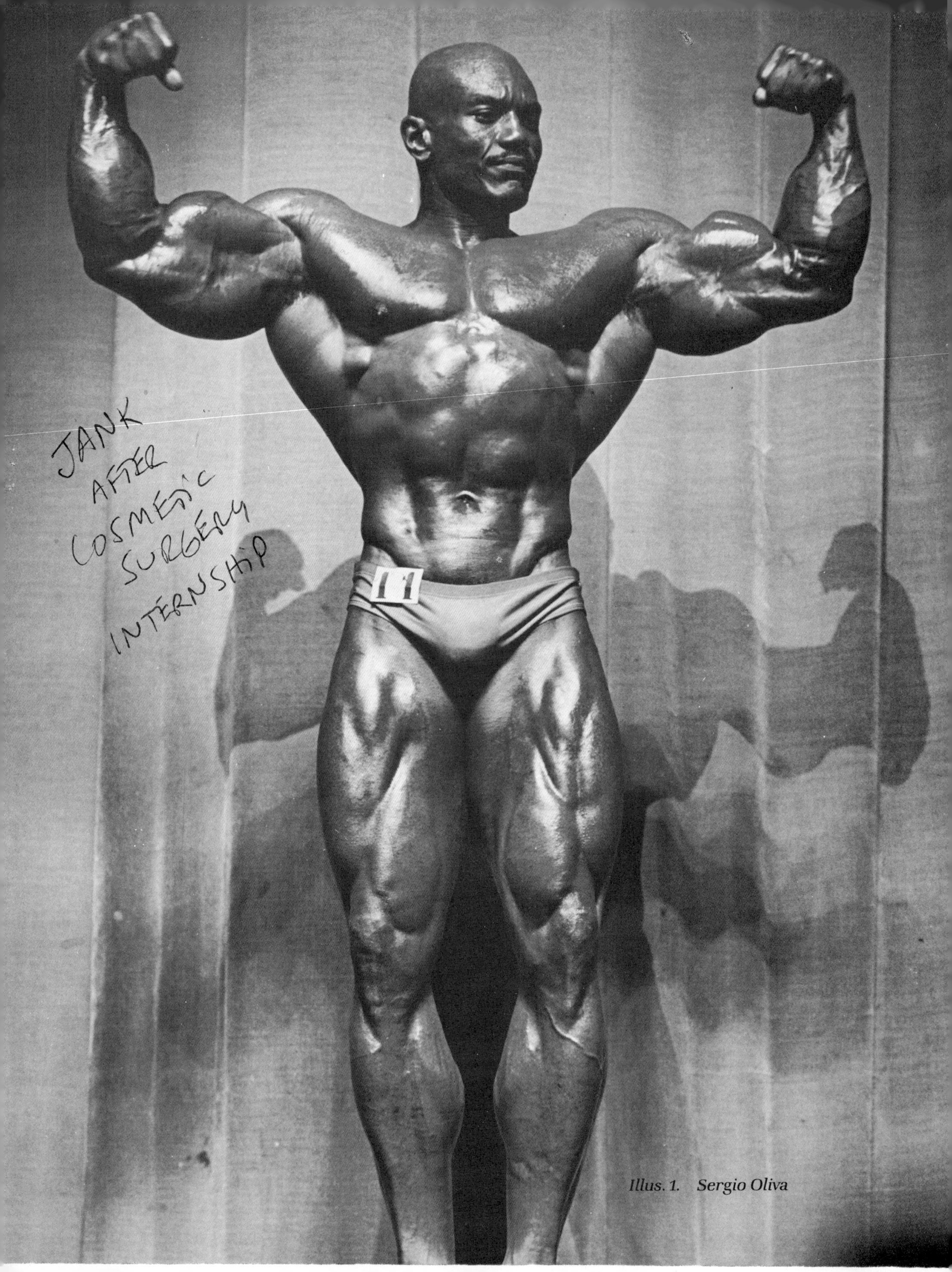

JANK
AFTER
COSMETIC
SURGERY
INTERNSHIP

Illus. 1.   Sergio Oliva

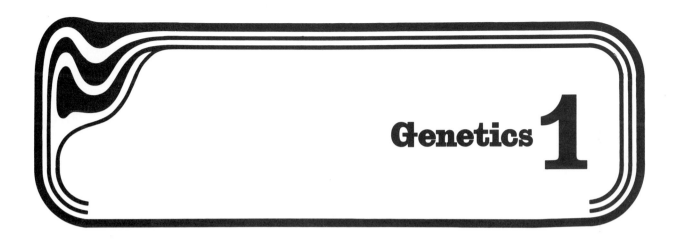

Genetics 1

The question on everyone's mind when first getting into bodybuilding, or even after many years in the sport, is: How good can I get? How defined? How big? How strong?

As you may have guessed, the answer is impossible to give with complete accuracy. Bodybuilding is not an exact science. For years it was a cult activity. Now it is considered a cross between a sport and an art, but a science it is *not*. No doubt in time bodybuilding will be studied systematically by scientists and answers found to some of the more difficult questions, but for the moment we have only a bit of knowledge to go on when rating someone's true potential.

Genetics is an important part of bodybuilding. Mr. Universe, Mike Mentzer, has often made the point that "choosing the right parents" is the surest way to bodybuilding success. All the rest is just following through on what nature bestowed upon you.

Thin bones often signify that a person cannot realistically expect to gain a huge amount of solid muscle. The ultimate limitation, however, is not the bones, but the muscle cells themselves. Arms and legs that even in the undeveloped person appear to have long, sweeping muscles are an indication of favorable genetics, and denote that an individual most likely possesses a full complement of muscle cells. We are all born with a different number, some

with literally millions more cells than others. Medical authorities tell us that this figure does not change during our lifetime. Bodybuilding or any other strenuous activity does not add muscle cells to your physique. It merely adds size to each cell. Strenuous activity plumps up each muscle cell so that it is better prepared to handle further demands.

It is not difficult to understand that if one man is born with three hundred thousand more cells in his upper arms than another, his potential for muscle building is accordingly far greater. Chances are the fellow who looks naturally well built has more than his share of cells. Alternately, the physically active man who still looks underdeveloped and frail probably has a small amount of cells. This does not mean that he can't develop good-looking 16-inch arms, 25-inch thighs and a 48-inch chest. It is just a pretty strong indication that he will not get into the 22-inch arm club now or in the future.

While bones do not necessarily tell the whole story, they are at least a pretty good indicator of potential in the majority of cases. A 6½-inch wrist or less is considered small, a 7-inch wrist is considered medium and above 7½ inches is regarded as large boned. With regular hard workouts most men should be able to obtain an upper arm measurement 10 inches above their wrist size. For example: A man with a 7-inch wrist should be able to obtain a 17-inch

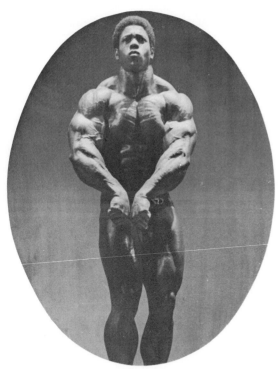

Illus. 2. Britain's Bertil Fox epitomizes what Hardcore Bodybuilding *is all about.*

muscular upper arm. As with everything, there are exceptions. French bodybuilder Serge Nubret has 21-inch arms and his wrists measure only 7-inches in circumference!

Another barometer of muscle-building potential, as difficult to estimate as muscle cell counts, is the amount of male hormone one possesses.

If you've ever watched boxing on TV, you have probably noticed that one of the fighters is more of a "natural" than the other: He looks stronger, more confident and has well-defined muscles. He's *loaded* with male hormones and is probably the more aggressive boxer, too. The other may have smoother lines, but be more timid. His male hormone count is lower, but he could still win the fight because his skill, reach and general stamina may be superior to the other fellow's. But that's boxing. It's different in bodybuilding. In our sport, having your fair share and more of male hormones is *vitally* important. Of course, many take male hormone drugs, testosterone and anabolic steroids, but that's another story.

Scientists are beginning to find out that male hormone production can be stimulated naturally by regular vigorous exercise (squats) and even by the sun. Regular, sensible sunbathing can possibly improve hormone production. Other practices, like the continued consumption of beer, lessen it.

Your progress in building muscular size and strength can also be limited by your pain threshold and your individual tolerance for physical exercise. If the words "hardy" and "rugged" fit an individual, that person likely has a high exercise tolerance and can recuperate quickly by the day after a heavy workout. On the other hand, if you are consistently tired and feel "out of sorts" after even moderate training, are suffering or shaking, or if you have diarrhea or a queasy stomach, you simply may not possess the constitution to endure the training needed to build a championship physique.

One interesting genetic characteristic is that you can be born with potential for building an impressive physique in only one part of your body and not in another. Many men, especially black men, have found that they have had enormous aptitude for building large arms or an imposing chest, yet building up the calves is, or appears to be, impossible. Because of inherited factors, the upper body contains a heroic supply of cellular potential, but the calves? They're little more than a small high knot of muscle that probably no amount of training could alter significantly.

Poor calf development is a trait of most but not *all* black men. Champion bodybuilders Chris Dickerson, Johnny Fuller, Bertil Fox and Sergio Oliva all have enormous lower leg development. They can thank their ancestors for giving them the cells to do the job.

Genetics, then, builds in your limitations. One small comfort is that as yet no one has utilized his physical potential to the full limits of his genetic capacity.

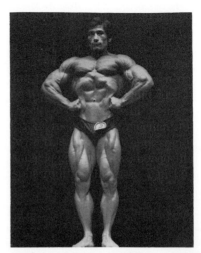

Illus. 3. Rochester's Danny Padilla—a "natural" if ever there was one.

Warming Up 2

Torn, sprained or strained muscles are painful and frustrating. At best they can make your training uncomfortable; at worst you could need an operation.

Most muscle strains repair themselves within days and sometimes training is not even halted. But there is reason to take care to prevent injury in the first place because it is unnecessary. You do not *have* to suffer a sore elbow, strained back or torn shoulder if you *warm up!*

There are three ways of warming up in bodybuilding. One is to warm up the overall physical motor—your heart, lungs and general circulation. Ideally, before embarking on a vigorous workout you should start with a few minutes of stretching, rope jumping or running in place. This will get your heart pumping strongly and your blood coursing through your veins. After that kind of warming up, you really feel like working out.

Stretching is extremely important in preventing and treating some weight-training injuries. Bodybuilders are not always sure which specific stretching exercises are best, though.

It is a good idea to perform the following miniroutine of stretching before beginning any exercises. Do them with smooth, gliding motions—do not bounce or tug doing any of them. Only those stretches that you repeat regularly will prove beneficial. All stretches should be done ten times, always holding the position till the count of ten.

If you find it difficult to perform any of these stretching movements, simply try your best and go through the motions. Your mobility will gradually improve, as will the effectiveness of your regular workout training. In a roundabout way stretching will help you get the most from your weights.

Stretch Exercise: Position #1

Adopt the lay-back position shown, gently stretching the frontal thigh muscles by bringing your ankle back to touch the back of your hips. Do not force the position or jerk the limbs. Follow the same procedure with the other leg.

Stretch Exercise: Position #2

Attempt to do a split, placing your legs as near as you can get to this position without straining. Place your hands on the floor to alleviate strain on the hamstrings.

Stretch Exercise: Position #3

Staying in the position adopted in the previous stretch, Position Two, attempt to slowly lower your head onto your knee, while also pulling your heel downward away from you.

A third—and equally important—form of warming up is doing at least one light warm-up set of each exercise before going on to attempt near-limit poundages for a certain number of repetitions

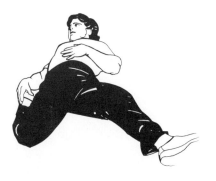

Position 1.

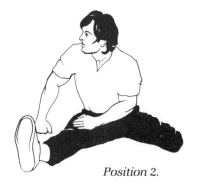

Position 2.

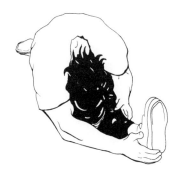

Position 3.

Illus. 4 - 6.   Stretching Exercise

(reps). This not only safeguards the muscles but also the tendons and joints. The human body is capable of incredible power and athletic performance, but it is an extremely sensitive and delicate machine, *especially* in a highly trained athlete, or an individual dedicated to pushing to new physical plateaus.

The irony is that your untrained brother, father, or mother may run for a bus or otherwise exert themselves, and suffer no after-effects from the effort. You, on the other hand, try the same thing and get a charley horse. Have you ever noticed champion runners suddenly pulling up with injuries during a race? The average *untrained* man, may not be as fast but he wouldn't have so many tears and sprains.

Why? Simply because a finely tuned engine such as your body in top training is more susceptible to the hazards of breakdown. The Lotus needs finer tuning and care than your average Ford. If it is not pampered and carefully tuned, it will not perform efficiently and if totally neglected, can even stop functioning.

As a bodybuilder, especially nearing peak condition, if you do not always warm up each body part thoroughly, you will sooner or later suffer a training injury which can set back your program anywhere from a few days to many months or even years.

Warm-ups become increasingly important as you gain size and strength. Warming up is also absolutely necessary for those who are getting on in years.

A famous bodybuilder who trained at the gym I frequented was such an enthusiast that if he was anywhere in the neighborhood he would have to pop in to chat with the guys. More often than not on these occasions, he would jump in on someone bench pressing and pound out as many reps as he could, without taking his jacket off! Several times he did this, completely cold, fully dressed: He'd jump in on the bench and pound out some reps, often with over 300 pounds. I could never understand how he could do it without warming up. Then one day . . . it happened. Rrr-ii-p! He tore his pectoral muscle from sternum to shoulder. After a lengthy recuperation period he was back in training, but with a difference. *Now* he warms up.

You should warm up with each exercise you do. If, for example, you normally barbell-curl 100 pounds for ten reps, then perform a set of ten to fifteen reps with about half that weight. A warm-up should not be so easy that the muscle is *not* stimulated to really work, nor on the other hand should it be so demanding as to pump up your muscles, spoiling them for the "quality" sets to come.

There is particular danger in changing exercises around. If, for example, you are used to performing overhead presses and lateral raises *prior* to heavy bench work, it would *not* be a good idea to suddenly perform the chest exercises *before* the shoulder routine. It could result in a nasty deltoid tear which would affect just about all your upper body training.

There are several really tricky moves in bodybuilding you have to watch out for: *Never* lift a loaded bar from the squat racks unless you are completely beneath it, both feet flat on the ground, evenly spaced, back flat.

Another no-no: Do not make a habit of regularly performing really heavy sets of barbell bent-over rowing. It's better to use a T–bar unit, or even safer, a single dumb-bell while propping up the body (and back) with your free hand on a bench. Seated single-arm curls can also cause a back problem. Beware of lifting too much weight.

Squats, especially if you lean too far forward, also can strain the lower back. Never bounce when in the full squat position. Merely lower slowly into the bent-knee position (thighs parallel to the floor) and rise quickly. Bouncing deeply could sooner or later wreck both your lower back *and* your knees.

Although relatively easy to avoid if good sense is used, training injuries are nevertheless very common. Eighty percent of all bodybuilders suffer a training injury within a twelve-month period. Fifteen percent are currently in the throes of an injury.

When you injure yourself the best thing to do is to apply ice to the immediate area as soon as possible. Cease all exercise and rest the area. The next day you may massage the area with your fingertips.

Be especially wary of returning to full-fledged exercise, and do not perform the movement which caused the injury in the first place. Never perform any exercise that causes even the slightest aggravation to your injury. This will worsen the strain. It is good to find an exercise that works the approximate area that *doesn't* cause pain.

As an example, assume you hurt your shoulder doing heavy bench presses (you didn't warm up sufficiently). You may find you cannot do flying exercises, bench presses or even incline bench work. But, glory be, there is no pain when you do decline bench presses. So rather than avoid all the chest exercises you should do decline bench presses. You will find that working *around* the injury in this way will actually help the recovery cycle and keep the muscle area toned up.

What is the most common cause of injury in bodybuilding? Egotism. So often a weight trainer

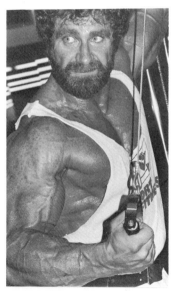

Illus. 7. Jusup Wilcosz warms up his triceps.

will be tempted to have a go at a weight that is far in excess of what he has done before. You may well be able to do flyes with 60-pound dumb-bells, but never be tempted to go for the "eighties" just because your workout partner can handle them with ease. Try "sixty fives," then "seventies." In due course you will get to the "eighties." It may take a while, but at least you'll get there injury-free.

The question of rupture or herniation often occurs to beginning weight trainers. Could it happen? Yes, but it's unlikely. I can recall only one of all the top bodybuilders ever rupturing himself while training. It is far more likely that you will rupture yourself by a sudden sneeze or cough than by following a regular regimen of pumping iron.

Workout Frequency 3

The more frequently you train, the faster your progress in bodybuilding—provided you fully recuperate (repair all broken-down muscle cells) after each workout. Experience has taught us that a muscle is not ready to be fully and progressively trained again before a 48-hour period. This may not apply to athletics, other sports activities or endurance skills, but it does apply to strenuous weight training. Weight training is the most arduous way to work the body's muscles known to man.

Beginners should train just three times a week, working the entire body at each training session, and resting at least one full day between workouts. The advanced or intermediate bodybuilder, however, often feels that training the whole body in one workout isn't practical. The beginner can do it easily because as a novice he will only be training with one or two sets per exercise and selecting just one movement for each muscle area.

But the more advanced trainer may want to perform more sets (three to five is average for the seasoned bodybuilder), and in most cases, he will opt to include two or three different exercises for each body part. You can readily see that this lengthens the workout considerably. Whereas the beginner will find he can complete his training in an hour or so, the experienced bodybuilder choosing to work each muscle for a longer duration and from a variety of

angles may find his workout time extending beyond three, four or even five hours. Not only does that mean he's practically living in the gym, having virtually no time for his wife and kids (or school work), but he may well find himself running out of steam, ultimately failing to complete the routine through utter exhaustion.

What is the solution? He must *split* his exercise schedule in two. (Some people even split their routines into three days.) The simplest way to divide your program is to save all upper body exercises for one training session and all lower body (leg) exercises for another. Alternatively, some bodybuilders like to do all pulling movements one day (rowing, curls, chins, etc.) and all pushing movements (presses, triceps, stretches and squats) another. My own preference is to work chest, back and arms one day and legs, shoulders and abdominals on the other days.

When you split a routine you can work out two successive days (or more) in a row because you are not working the same muscles each day. One day you may be working the chest and legs, and the next day the back and arms will come in for the onslaught. Your recuperative mechanism can generally cope with this. What it cannot stand is working the same muscle group on two consecutive days.

The split routine therefore can be performed

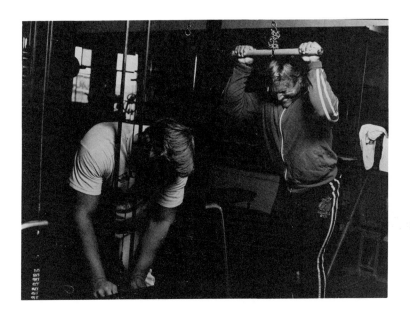

Illus. 8.   Popular muscular marvel Tom Platz is famous for being an immensely hard trainer. The severity of his workouts puts other bodybuilders in the shade.

four days a week (working each body part twice a week), or you may take six workouts a week (training each body area three times weekly). This latter plan is usually adopted by bodybuilders six or eight weeks before a contest. To train six days a week all year round is often too much work and can cause overtraining or burning out. Your gains can come to a standstill, or worse, you could actually start *losing* size and strength. For short-term (precontest) training, however, the six-day split method is very popular, as it can lead to a spurt of added size and increased muscularity.

A very workable (and increasingly popular) method of training is the *every-other-day split*, in which you perform half your workout one day followed by complete rest the day after. On the day after your rest day, train the other half of your body and rest again the next day. Obviously, this does not fit neatly into the 7 day weekly cycle: It is strictly for home trainers who have access to their own gyms any day of the week or for gym trainers whose commercial gym is open all week long.

Florida bodybuilding star Frank Calta has his own version of the every-other-day split which he calls "rotation for recuperation."

According to this principle, you train just three days a week (usually Monday, Wednesday and Friday), but split the workout into two fairly equal halves. However, unlike the every-other-day-split routine, Calta's method allows you a two-day rest on weekends. The every-other-day split method never

gives you more than one day off at a time. Calta's rotation principle is compatible with strongman Fred Howell's belief: "The less you train, the more you gain." Naturally Howell, who has been given the unofficial title of "World's Strongest Home Trainer," does not mean his slogan to be taken too literally, but he does genuinely feel that most iron men train too long and far too frequently.

Arnold Schwarzenegger has seemingly proved that one can train *twice* a day, *six* days a week and make progress in size and shape, but even the "Austrian Oak" could only do this for a limited time prior to an upcoming contest. His usual practice was to work out less frequently.

Apart from their very real dangers, artificial steroids are believed to add greatly to one's recuperative powers, and may be one reason why certain bodybuilders can often train every day and make gains while others simply must have rest days or else quickly become stale from overtraining.

Training frequency is a vital factor in your bodybuilding success. Obviously if you are going to take the kind of five- and six-hour workouts Pete Grymkowski, Steve Michalik and Roy Callender have become famous for, you will need your recuperation days of total abstinence from the iron. Short workouts, however, may allow you more frequent training. Tailor your workout frequency to your individual constitution, and if you are enjoying the pumping iron adventure, and, more importantly, growing from it, your exercise frequency is on target. Keep it up!

Sets and Reps 4

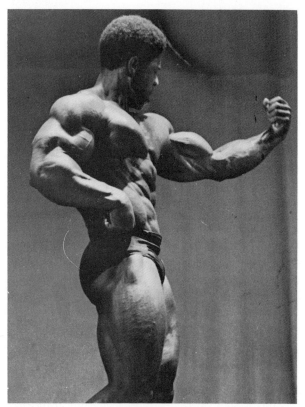

Illus. 9.   *Bertil Fox trains heavy, long, and hard—he seldom uses high reps and light weights.*

The question of the optimum number of sets and reps is on most bodybuilders' minds most of the time. A bodybuilder wants to reach his or her objective as quickly as possible and can't afford to waste time. If he isn't using the correct reps/sets formula, all that hard training will have been in vain.

There is no exact system of sets and reps, no "average" that *always* works. I would guess that the average number of sets per exercise would be about four, while the average number of reps would be eight or nine—the average, if adopted in *your* routine will not necessarily give *you* positive results.

Johnny Fuller, that awesome British bodybuilder, is successful with a system whereby he performs 10 sets of 32 repetitions of each exercise. He actually finds this to be the most workable of all the systems he has tried over some 25 years.

In contrast, Mike Mentzer promotes the use of only 1 or 2 sets of an exercise, with 10 to 12 repetitions.

Arnold Schwarzenegger, however, contends that a system of at least 20 sets per body part (which can include 4 different exercises for that part, 5 sets per exercise) is best for advanced training gains.

The curious thing is that many established stars built their bodies with a variety of set and rep permutations, quite often opting for lower, heavier repetitions during their early years, and invariably selecting higher, lighter and more pump-oriented repetitions during the latter part of their careers.

Witness Reg Park. Reg preferred performing 10 or 12 reps of each exercise, up until winning the 1951 N.A.B.B.A. Mr. Universe Contest. Subsequently he added further size and, of course, strength by adopting a system of using only five repetitions per set (and up to eight sets). This enabled him to obtain his maximum size for the period until his 1958 N.A.B.B.A. Mr. Universe win after which he again, with some initial difficulty, practiced higher repetitions (10) and gained even more size. Why was it difficult? By Reg's own account he had gotten used to performing the lower reps which did not tax his stamina, only his tendons and ligaments. Consequently when the higher reps were introduced, he had enormous lactic acid buildup in the muscles and found the higher reps far more difficult to perform even though considerably less poundage was being used.

Arnold, too, spent his early workouts using heavy weights and low reps. He had 18-inch arms at the age of 18, 20-inch arms at the age of 19 and whopping 22-inch arms at the tender age of 20. The Austrian could also deadlift 600 pounds, bench press 400, squat 500 and curl a mammoth 280.

After building his huge body with heavy weights and winning several Mr. Universe titles along the way, Arnold came to California, the mecca of world bodybuilding, and for the most part used higher reps. This gave him a little more size, and along with an improved diet, helped in making him extremely muscular and defined. Arnold's reps at this time were around 10, but for his lower body, he would push the reps even higher—he did 12 to 15. His legs improved dramatically.

Bill Pearl, another giant of the '60s and '70s, also performed low and high reps. He would work at the weights using a system of 5 repetitions, or as many as 12, combining at times both systems—not, it may be noted, by performing an average 8 or 9 reps, but choosing to perform sets of either high or low repetitions.

Is there a lesson here? Are the moderate repetitions worth less? No, because many successful bodybuilders have made their mark training using around eight reps per set. My own conclusion, however, is that moderate repetitions are the least beneficial to the bodybuilder. I feel that tendon, ligament and basic muscle fibre are stimulated directly by using four to six reps, while capillary stimulation and "pump" come from twelve or more. Certainly it is hard to get a heavy pump from fewer than ten reps. True, a "burn" isn't everything, but it helps when you want to shock your muscles out of complacency and force blood into the area being trained.

Many bodybuilders, especially those from the old physical culture (p.c.) school, have a revulsion for today's bodybuilding training, especially the terminology used in some of the muscle magazines. Such sayings as "cutting up," "super-sets," "blitz," "bomb" and "giant-sets" disgust them. "Whatever happened to good old p.c.," they cry, "when after a workout a bodybuilder would perform some gymnastics, maybe practice a little judo or weightlifting form, and then dive into an ice cold sea?" Among the expressions that cause particular irritation to the p.c. brigade is "breaking the pain barrier."

To a man, these p.c. disciples, bless 'em, abhor the thought. "After all," they argue, "in the old days we took tough workouts and really lifted pretty hard, but now these modern pumpers talk about 'breaking the pain barrier' . . . no pain, no gain. It's unbelievable."

There is evidence to show that the intermediate or advanced bodybuilder who is prepared to blast through the pain (or burn) that comes on or about the twelfth rep will stand an improved chance of building bigger muscles at a faster rate than if he chose to end the set the moment the burning started.

Bodybuilding writer Norman Zale wrote me recently that the YMCA gym in Chicago now has 15,000 paid-up members, many of whom are following the heavy-duty system of maximum effort and minimum

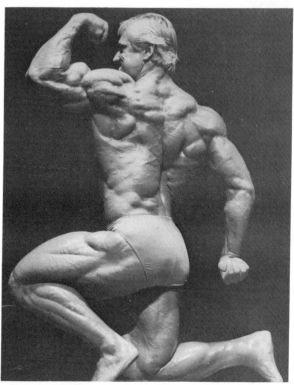

Illus. 10.   Each set that Tom Platz performs is of supreme quality. It is doubtful that any of his workouts is less than perfect.

(one or two) sets. "They are performing all kinds of 'negatives' and 'forced reps,'" he writes, "but the fellows who are making the gains are the guys who are performing three or four exercises per body part, four or five sets each, ten to twelve reps. The heavy duty advocates, and there are plenty of them, are, as a rule, not growing. . . ."

In a letter I published in my magazine, *Muscle-Mag International*, from Mario Savva, an English reader, Zale's opinion was confirmed: "The people who advocate low sets and heavy weights, like Mike Mentzer, base this method of training on the fact that its effect is more intense than the 20 sets per body part commonly used by bodybuilders. Their arguments are logical and would be the final word on the subject, but for the simple fact that *intensity* of exercise is not the only factor in developing muscle.

The muscle which bodybuilders develop and display has three constituents, apart from fat and water: red, slow-twitch muscle fibres; white, fast-twitch muscle fibres and blood capillaries. Heavy-duty training, like powerlifting and weightlifting, develops mainly fast-twitch fibres (which are used for anaerobic, high-strength work as opposed to slow-twitch fibres which are used for aerobic, low-strength work) leaving slow-twitch fibres and blood capillaries underdeveloped.

Mario Savva goes on to note that strong men often do not have big muscles, so Mentzer cannot just dismiss the phenomenon as purely genetic variations among people. Big muscles—big by body-building standards—are not a prerequisite for weightlifting, powerlifting, shot-putting, discus, or javelin-throwing. These are all power events of *short* duration. But when one looks at sports such as bodybuilding, gymnastics or boxing in which training is based on power, strength and *endurance*, then big muscles are generally the rule. Boxing is not so clear-cut a case, but there are good examples such as Ken Norton and Mike Weaver.

Bodybuilders who train 20 sets per body part create sufficient intensity to develop fast-twitch muscle fibres, but also, because of the duration, develop slow-twitch fibres and blood capillaries. Therefore the pump does have some practical use.

This hypothesis is the only one truly consistent with what occurs in reality. The best bodybuilders of the last 30 years have all done around 20 sets per body part. The greatest two, Sergio Oliva and Arnold Schwarzenegger, generally do five sets per exercise and Serge Nubret does about eight to ten. Roy Callender spends up to *seven* hours in the gym.

How many sets and reps do other champs perform? According to George Snyder's and Rick Wayne's *3 More Reps!* series, the most credible training books on the market, here are some other champs' choices: Bill Grant appears to favor 5 sets of 12 reps; Ken Waller likes 4 sets of 12 reps; Dave Draper, 5 sets of 10–12 reps; Leroy Colbert, 6 sets of 12 reps; Franco Columbu, 4–5 sets of 10 reps; Rocky De Ferro, 3 sets of 10 reps and Ron Teufel, 5 sets of 12–15 reps.

Of course, very few champs keep their systems unchanged. Many times they will alter them for variety. Also, it is interesting to note that most body-building stars train their legs and abdominals with higher repetitions than they use for other body parts.

It is quite common for a bodybuilder to perform sets of 6 reps in the press and bench press only to jump to 15 reps for thigh training and 20 repetitions or more for calf and abdominal training. Forearms, too, are a popular target for higher repetitions.

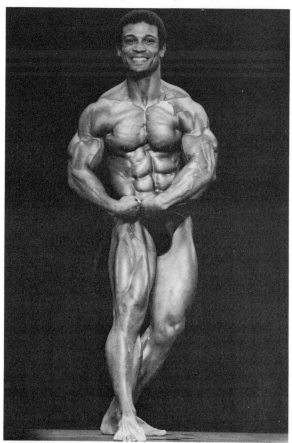

Illus. 11. Mohamed Makkawy exercises in perfect style, using moderate weights. Super-heavy weights and low reps are not part of his present training.

Savva comments that although Mentzer feels that one overtrains using 20 sets per body part, in fact 20 sets can be as exhausting or nonexhausting as you like, depending entirely on the amount of weight you use. Obviously, if you try to push to failure on each set, you are asking for trouble, but if you only go to failure on the last set of an exercise, there is less danger of overtraining.

Despite these critical remarks about heavy duty, a lot of what Mike Mentzer says makes sense. I believe that your genetic potential can be realized after you reach a plateau (which is not due to overtraining) by changing your training continually to and from, say, ten sets per exercise to four to five sets per exercise to heavy duty to basic powerlifting.

Hypertrophy is a big concern of bodybuilders trying to increase muscle mass. It is not the same thing as a gain in strength and occurs when the muscle is sufficiently overloaded and there's a certain leap in the supply of blood to the muscle. The pump plays its part in this growth of muscle size.

In an excellent article in *Muscle and Fitness* magazine (September 1980), "How to Build Muscle," Dr. Gold has pointed out that if you train with single reps the way some powerlifters do, you get stronger than the average bodybuilder who is doing eight or ten reps per set. But this strength only applies to doing one rep, and you will probably gain less muscle mass than by training with additional reps. Runners or swimmers, whose activities are highly repetitive, do not build massive muscles as a rule because they do not overload their muscles in their workouts. "It takes the combination of muscular overload plus additional blood flow to the muscles to create the kind of hypertrophy that bodybuilders want," Dr. Gold advises.

Finally, Savva reminds us, a bodybuilder can have large well-defined muscles because of an expansion of blood vessels rather than an expansion of muscle fibres.

Steve Reeves, the handsome "Hercules" of movie fame, was a legend in the bodybuilding game, possessing extremely well-formed muscles. He worked hard using a system of 12 to 15 reps per set. Occasionally, feeling the need for a heavy workout, he would drop the reps down somewhat, but it would be fair to say that Steve was a product of hard training . . . high rep training.

Ironically, he was known for his unwillingness to stop a particular set. Typical of Reeves would be the instance where he had worked a curl to maximum, and unable to complete the movement by bi-

ceps power, he would help the dumb-bell up by lifting it with his foot or the free hand, only to lower it slowly under stress (negatives).

Now almost forty years later, Mr. Universe Tom Platz does something similar. He just keeps his sets going (up to five minutes) and when unable to perform a complete movement, he will do "partials" or merely rock the weight back and forth to keep the burn in the muscle for that little bit longer. In the upright rowing exercise Tom will do eight or ten complete reps, pulling the weight all the way from a straight-arm-hang to his chin. As his shoulders and limbs eventually tire, he will only be able to raise the weight partially. Rather than stop the exercise at this point, Platz will continue to try to lift the barbell. He will rock it up and down, keeping the burn in the muscles as long as possible. If he can get some movement from an exercise, then that exercise is not finished. Only when there is absolutely no movement will Platz "call it a day" and admit that the set is finished.

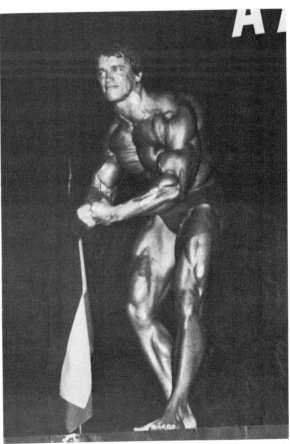

Illus. 12. Early on in his career Arnold used extremely heavy weights and low reps; later he turned to more moderate weights and higher reps.

Breathing 5

Proper breathing is particularly important during exercise, especially vigorous exercise such as weight training. One of the biggest misconceptions is that during exercise you should breathe in through the nose and out through the mouth. This is nonsense. There are times when the trainer may be able to breathe in through the nose, usually during slow nonstrenuous exercise, but for the most part, you will need to inhale through your mouth.

Each bodybuilding exercise has its own tailor-made breathing pattern which you will learn in time. Generally, you can apply the following rule as a rough guide. Inhale during the easiest part of the exercise and exhale just as you complete the hardest part. For example, in the squat, gulp air prior to squatting down into the bent-knee position and exhale just as you straighten up again.

You may find that in the most exertive exercises, especially as the reps begin to get tough, it helps to expel the air aggressively like a piston at the conclusion of each rep.

Also, on the most vigorous movements, you may take several breaths between the last few reps if oxygen seems to be required.

Deep breathing can act as a pacer for your repetitions. For the most part one breath per rep will help keep your rhythm during an exercise.

I am continually surprised by the advice some writers give to bodybuilders on breathing. One expert who should know better writes: "The most important thing to remember is never hold your breath while lifting." This is absolute nonsense. I would like to see that author come out of a heavy squat without holding his breath.

Another writer, a Mr. Olympia winner, in his book concludes that you should always breathe in through your nose when exercising with or without weights ". . . to purify the air before it reaches the lungs." I suggest this man try breathing through his nose the next time he completes a set of squats or bench presses or runs a marathon.

This kind of advice is invariably the result of champion bodybuilders using ghost writers—often men or women who have very little idea about what hardcore bodybuilding is all about. They write on what they *feel* is correct breathing and the star bodybuilder in question doesn't bother to correct the statement when and if he reads what he is supposed to have written.

You should always have plenty of oxygen when you exercise. Many bodybuilders like to train out-of-doors for this reason, at least part of the year. I feel that outdoor gym areas will become more popular in the next decade.

Remember that a good oxygen supply keeps your energy level up and enables you to train longer and harder without exhaustion.

The Perfect Set 6

Time is short. Before you know it the game is over. Young, middle-aged or old, you will one day find that your time has mysteriously run out. You will regret it deeply and wonder where it went.

Do not waste time. In bodybuilding it is an easy thing to do. You may go from workout to workout, pretending to be doing the right thing, yet in reality you are wasting your exercise sessions. A training workout is of no use unless it is productive. If you have made no improvements over the last year of training, then that is a year *out* of your bodybuilding life—twelve months wasted. Not, by any means, the way to championship muscles.

Each workout, each set performed in that workout, must contribute to positive results. Frank Zane, three-time Mr. Olympia, recalls: "I will never forget training at Gold's one day prior to an important contest. I was training my triceps and had worked up a really good pump. I had practically blanked out my surroundings from my mind. Then John Balik came into the gym to tell me something important, and I interrupted my workout for a few seconds. I could have kicked myself afterwards for taking the time to talk to John. In the few seconds that I took my mind off what I was doing I lost all my concentration, and I lost my pump. No matter how hard I tried I just couldn't get that pumped-up feeling back. My whole workout was spoiled that day. So you have to keep your mind on your training once you get going in the

gym. Let everything else wait. The gym is no place to conduct business or pleasure. You go there only to train with 100 percent concentration. Make every set count. Work for a greater pump each set."

Time may be on your side now. Keep ahead of the game. Make each workout a positive, useful experience. This attitude will lead to success.

What is the perfect set? It begins with an attitude of mind; don't even begin a set unless you are ready for it mentally. Olympic and powerlifters take time to ready themselves for a lift. In the same way

Illus. 13.   Intensity and concentration make Tony Emmott's sets top quality.

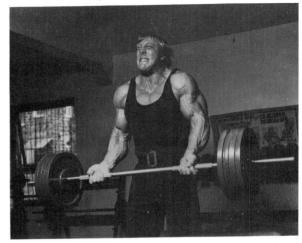

19

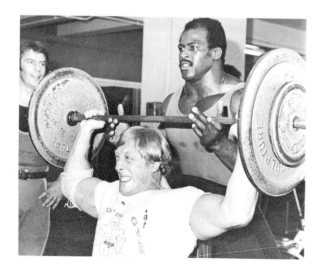

Illus. 14.   Training with a partner can be very beneficial. Tony Emmott and Bill Richardson show how.

you must zero in on *your* set. You cannot expect to be joking around one minute and then throw yourself into a perfect set. It doesn't work that way. You must will yourself into the correct frame of mind. Bronston Austin, a strong candidate for high physique honors in the near future, openly groans during his pre-set psyching. A little melodramatic? Perhaps, but it works for him. Few people can give their all to each set like Bronston.

Roy Callender is another who psychs up for a few seconds prior to performing a set. It's as though he's confirming in his mind the exact rep target he's going to achieve.

Another factor in quality training is the environment. You just cannot do justice to your workout if you are training with others who are not dedicated to progressive bodybuilding. Jokers will turn your workout into a joke. Neither do you want a training partner who yells and screams at you to complete a set.

Arnold Schwarzenegger has always chosen workout partners—Draper, Corney, Columbu, Wilcosz—who are dedicated to their training. In turn he gives quiet but meaningful encouragement during *their* sets. Typical of the big Austrian, he will lean forward during a set of bench presses and almost whisper, "One more, Franco. . . ." This *encourages* much more than a huge cavalcade of shouts and screams.

Every set you do should at least start off in perfect style. Sometimes allowing a looseness to take over can be beneficial, but generally speaking you should try to maintain good form. Concentrate intensely as the rep count goes up. Do not allow outside or negative thoughts to penetrate your mind. Be determined first to target and then achieve your goal. If you have set your mind on eight reps, then that is what you must do.

Although forced and negative reps need not be a part of every set it can certainly be beneficial to perform some as your set is completed. Your training partner must be in tune with your every move and need: If you have to waste energy directing him what to do, the set will be pretty well shot.

Another positive aid to the effectiveness of your set is active visualization . . . seeing your muscles bursting with added size . . . believing in their instant growth. It works!

Squeezing the muscles at the "top" of each rep can give even more value to the set. Burns, short quick reps (usually three or four) can prove helpful by isolating the action, and intensifying the pain for extra effectiveness. Ask Larry Scott about burns. Better yet, look at his 21-inch arms!

When a set is finally over, try to hold onto the bar, squeeze it for a second or two and let go slowly.

When it's your turn to rest between sets use that rest period. Sit and concentrate Never allow your mind to get led away between sets, or get drawn into conversation. Do not answer phones, meet new people, sing to the radio, watch television or go to the washroom. The time for any break or relaxation is after working a particular body part. Then, and only then, can you take five . . . or ten, if you like.

Beginner's Game Plan 7

Most of this book deals with bodybuilding on a more advanced level. However, every day we see an influx of hundreds, perhaps thousands of newcomers to the sport, a number of whom may choose to beg, borrow or steal this book. If you are a beginner to bodybuilding, there is one thing I know for sure: *You* are confused!

I have noted that bodybuilding is *not* an exact science. It's still pretty much a hit and miss affair, at least for most of its fledgling trainers. Much of the problem comes from the reams of conflicting advice available on the subject. Not only will you read of different rules in bodybuilding, but you may well see them in the same magazine. As is often the case, the most rigid opinions are held by those with the least knowledge. True, rules are made to be broken, but there *are* basic "do's" and "don'ts" which if followed will give you the best chance of success.

Beginners seek the fastest, surest and safest way to build muscle size, strength, vigorous health and well-being. Often, going at it on their own or taking bad advice (firsthand or in print), they achieve virtually the opposite effect. Their training progress is slowed or nonexistent, and they end up tired and disenchanted with the whole scene—often giving up in disgust at not being able to succeed.

Remember the shortest route is the correct route. If you choose the wrong path at the beginning of your journey, you may never get to your destination.

Bodybuilding for the beginner must be simple. It should involve workouts which are relatively short so that sufficient recuperative time is allowed between workouts to get the torn-down cells repaired. You must eat well regularly and get adequate or more than adequate sleep.

So there you have it: exercise, food, rest. Get them right and you are on your way.

The principles I am laying down are not the last word: There is always room for various ideas and differing opinions. I suggest, however, that you stick to my advice here at least in the beginning, and don't allow yourself to be influenced by what others say or by whatever else you may read, or you may become quite confused. Even if other ideas are also workable, chopping and changing them at the embryo stage is not advised. You may even find articles in old bodybuilding magazines or books that I have written which differ from my present advice. Pay them no heed. Stay on track with me *now* and your initiation into the iron game will be relatively problem-free.

The first thing a beginner must do is get a checkup from his doctor. Ask for a stress test and a complete physical examination and tell him you are taking up a program of vigorous bodybuilding. If he can't do it in his office he will arrange for you to be tested at another office. You will be asked to step up and down on a bench, jog on a machine or ride a stationary bike while your heart is monitored. The test is nothing to worry about. It can even be fun, and chances are he'll be pleased that you have chosen to enter into healthful, vigorous exercise. The reason I ask you to go for a complete checkup is that if by chance you had a heart or other organic problem, you could worsen the condition with heavy exercise. Far better to have it detected so that the doctor can recommend treatment than risk further aggravation by plunging into a strenuous routine without having a clean bill of health.

Bodybuilding is an athletic pursuit and you have to be in robust health to benefit from the training. If you are over forty years of age, a complete stress test is even more necessary. And if you have been a heavy drinker and smoker since your teens and have not exercised formally since your school years, I suggest you clean up your act now, before even going for that stress test.

Your exercise program consists of just eight movements. These are all you perform. Do not add exercises of your own. Do not change the order of the exercises listed. Do not leave out movements, nor increase your training days. If you feel that your arms (or legs or chest, etc.) are extra-skinny and need more work, do not add additional movements for these areas. Keep to what I say, and only what I say.

At the end of this chapter, I describe the eight exercises that constitute the beginner's game plan. Each exercise is to be performed in just one "set" of eight to ten repetitions. That means you do only one series of eight to ten counts. Pushing a barbell up/down is one count, doing it again is two counts, and so on. In the sport of bodybuilding an up/down movement with a weight is known as a *repetition*. If you do, say, one series of eight repetitions, this is known as one set of eight reps (written: 1 × 8). If after putting the weight down and resting for a minute or two you do another series of eight repetitions, this is known as two sets of eight reps (written: 2 × 8) and so on. Some advanced bodybuilders perform up to ten sets on just one exercise, but the usual figure is between three and five. You, as a beginner, are hereby instructed to do just one set, for the time being.

The set you do must contain eight repetitions (except the calves and abdominals. Do 12 to 25 reps for these two areas.) As you advance from workout to workout you will notice that the weight starts to feel different—lighter. It hasn't lost any poundage of course. *YOU* are the agent responsible for this phenomenon. Your strength has increased. After a cou-

ple of workouts you will find that you are able to do more repetitions without undue strain—do them! When you reach 12, add more weight to the bar, not an excessive amount, but just enough to allow you to achieve your original eight repetitions. Plug away until again after a few more workouts you have achieved 12 full and unstrained repetitions. It is important to apply your mental and physical effort to improving the number of reps you attain, but never do this to the extent of "throwing" the weight up or "leaning back" excessively during the movement. This is called loose style or cheating and has no place in a beginner's program. Controlled cheating is another matter. It is an advanced principle (see Chapter 23 on principles and techniques) which can be applied when you are beyond the beginner's stage of bodybuilding and well on the way up the ladder to bigger and better things.

The number of days you train (training frequency) has a lot to do with your progress. As a beginner you must train three times a week, exercising the entire body—torso, back, arms and legs—each session, having at least a day's rest between each workout. Most find that training Mondays, Wednesdays and Fridays is ideal, leaving the weekend free. Do not be tempted to work out more frequently. It could easily lead to overtraining and reverse your progress. Remember, even the most advanced bodybuilders do not train each body part more than three times a week. (What they often do is "split" their routine in two and exercise six days a week, but that is still not working each body part more frequently.) Needless to say, six-day-a-week training is not for the beginner. You need that day's rest between workouts to fully recuperate. Even advanced bodybuilders with superbly conditioned bodies often only go to six-day-a-week training to temporarily sharpen up for a contest.

For a bodybuilder—especially the beginner—eating habits directly translate into progress, or lack of it. You are indeed a result of what you eat. If you are excruciatingly skinny, you will need to increase your overall calorie intake. This can be done by eating bigger meals, but it is usually best brought about by eating more frequent, if smaller, meals.

Milk is the world's number one weight gaining product. Drink plenty of it whenever you can, whole, skimmed or partly skimmed.

Every meal should contain at least some high protein food such as cheese, eggs, milk, meat, nuts, poultry or fish. Balance out your eating with fresh fruits, peas, beans, potatoes, brown rice and other grains, leafy greens, salads, whole grain cereals, and whole wheat bread.

Try to steer clear of sugar-loaded soft drinks, cakes, cookies, candies and *all* foods to which sugar is unnecessarily added. Turn your nose up at all the artificial, cellophane-wrapped, icing-coated junk food that fills the store today. They are garbage and will turn your system into nothing but a garbage dump.

When first getting into bodybuilding you must make sure that you get adequate sleep and rest: seven, eight or nine hours, depending on your needs. It is far better to get a regular eight hours sleep each night than go with only a few hours for several nights and then try to "make up" the sleep by staying in bed most of the weekend. Wild partying (and the smoking and drinking that often go with it) are most definitely *not* conducive to making rapid bodybuilding gains.

Gains in muscle size and strength come quickly for the beginner. Of course they will *never* come quickly enough for you, but you will be pleasantly surprised if you keep up your training. Don't *expect* overnight results, and when after a few months you have gained a significant amount of body weight and muscle size, in retrospect the results will seem to have arrived overnight.

More does not mean *better* at the beginner's stage. The beginner's exercises, to be performed in order, are one set of eight reps of each of the following:

1. *Press behind Neck*
2. *Squat*
3. *Bench Press*
4. *Wide-Grip Chins*
5. *Barbell Curl*
6. *Lying Triceps Extension*
7. *Standing Calf Raise*
8. *Crunches*

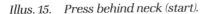

1. Press behind Neck

This is probably the all-time most popular movement for size building. The lateral (side) head of the deltoid is worked most, although all three areas are exercised. Perform eight to ten repetitions with a barbell weighing 40 to 50 pounds. Inhale before pushing up and exhale as the arms lock out.

When you get to the stage of being able to handle fairly hefty weights (about 130 pounds) you may take the weight from squat racks to make it easier to get to the initial behind-the-neck position. Some

bodybuilders prefer to perform this exercise in the seated position. This eliminates any help that you might sometimes unconsciously use in the lift. Grip the bar so that your forearms can be vertical when the weight is resting on your shoulders. Perform your reps without pausing, and keep your back straight during the exercise. Although primarily a shoulder exercise, this movement also works the upper back, the *trapezius* and the *triceps* of the upper arm.

Illus. 15.   Press behind neck (start).

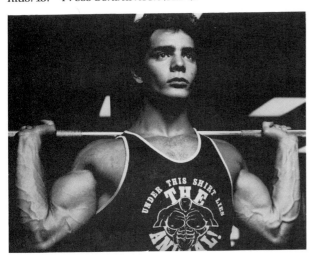

Illus. 16.   Press behind neck (finish).

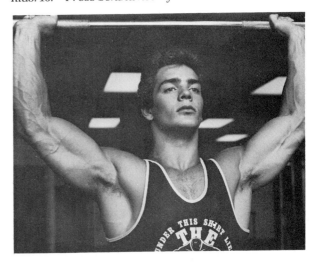

2. Squat

The regular barbell squat is like the free-standing squat, with the addition of a loaded barbell across the back of your shoulders. It is very good for the quadriceps. If you are very underweight, you may want to wrap a towel around the bar where it rests on the upper back to help prevent the bar from chafing your skin. It is important to keep your head up and your back flat during the entire movement. Starting poundages vary from 50 to 100 pounds depending on your present strength and condition. Many bodybuilders are able to squat with double their body weight. The best squatter of all time was Paul Anderson who, at 400 pounds, squatted once with 1,230 pounds!

One interesting aspect of squatting is that regular heavy squatting (say five sets of ten reps) puts such demands on the system that invariably the metabolism reacts and growth of the entire body is stimulated. Some authorities actually claim that squatting causes the body to manufacture far more of its own natural steroids.

Whatever the case, squats are responsible for more muscle growth than any other single exercise.

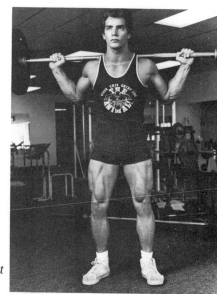

Illus. 17. Squat (start).

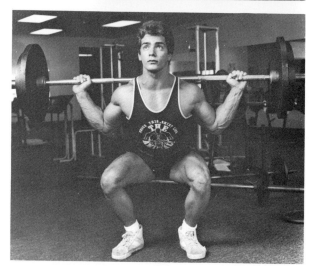

Illus. 18.   Squat (finish).

3. Bench Press

It doesn't take a genius to see that the bench press movement is in fact an upside-down floor dip. But it is superior as a chest-building exercise because you do not have to hold your body straight, nor do you have to balance to the same extent. The most important factor is that you can add small amounts of weight to the bar on a regular basis. In this way the movement uses progressive resistance to build muscle steadily. Before you know it, you'll be handling respectable poundage in this exercise. Start with 40 to 60 pounds, and be prepared to handle 200 pounds or more within your first year of training. Inhale as you lower the weight; exhale as it goes up. (Imagine you are blowing it up.) Most peo-

ple lower the weight to the nipple area, but those who wish to build "higher" pectorals may lower the bar to the upper chest. Under no circumstances allow the weight to bounce from the sternum (chest bone) as this could damage the delicate nerve center located beneath it.

When bench-pressing, grip so that the forearms are vertical when the bar is resting on the chest. Push the weight up to arm's length. Do not allow the weight to drop, but rather lower it with control to the original position. Perform between 4 to 15 reps. (Strength comes from 4 to 5 reps; muscle size comes from 6 to 15.) The bench press has been nicknamed the king of the torso builders because of the growth-producing effect it has on the entire upper body.

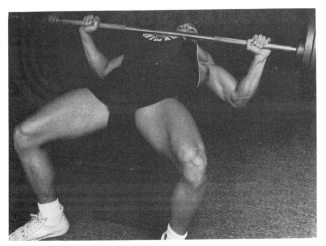

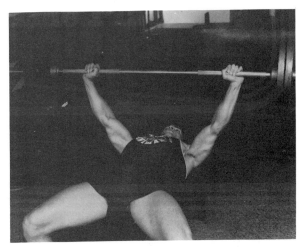

Illus. 19. Bench press (start).   *Illus. 20. Bench press (finish).*

4. Wide-Grip Chins

A very important bodybuilding exercise, wide grip chins are performed by just about every bodybuilding champion. Start by hanging from a high horizontal chin bar. Make sure that the lats are fully stretched and the arms are straight. Pull up strongly (keeping the elbows back) until the bar is behind your head. Lower and repeat. If you try to "concentrate" the effort into your lats, they will benefit. At first you may find this exercise difficult to perform.

Keep persevering. Aim ultimately for 12 to 15 reps even though at first you may only be able to perform one or two reps. Inhale before raising up and exhale as the bar arrives behind your head.

The great benefit offered by this exercise is a wider back. There is a tendency for the *scapula* (shoulder blade) to be pulled outward. There is also a long-term benefit to your shoulder width. In fact the wide-grip chin helps lift the entire upper body.

Illus. 21. Wide-grip chins (start).   *Illus. 22. Wide-grip chins (finish).*

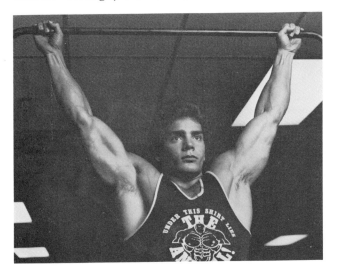

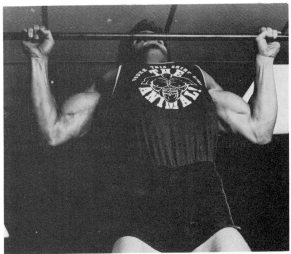

5. Barbell Curl

Stand with legs comfortably apart, holding a barbell loaded to about 40 pounds. Your grip should be about shoulder-width, or perhaps slightly wider. Without leaning back, take a deep breath and "curl" the barbell to the shoulders. Do not bend the knees; try to raise the weight while keeping your elbows fairly close to your body. Exhale as the bar arrives at your shoulder level; lower at the same speed at which you raised it, and repeat. Try for 10 repetitions. This is the most basic of all biceps exercises and is the best one for building up that muscle.

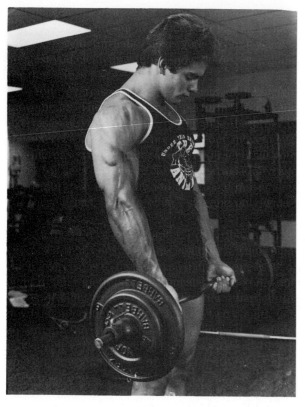

Illus. 23.   Barbell curl (start).

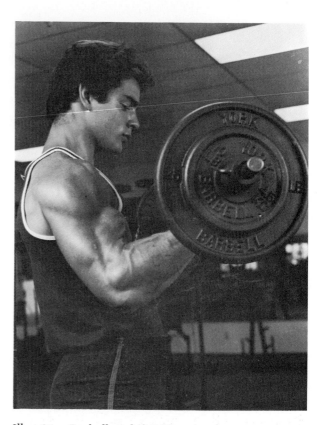

Illus. 24.   Barbell curl (finish).

6. Lying Triceps Extension

This exercise builds more size into the triceps than any other single movement. Lie on a flat bench, holding a moderately weighted barbell, with your hands from 2 to 10 inches apart. Keeping the upper arms vertical, raise the barbell up and down behind the head. Inhale before the lift. Exhale as the arms straighten. Try 8 to 10 reps.

7. Standing Calf Raise

This exercise gives the calves a good workout. It involves the simple process of rising up on your toes (lifting the heels). The resistance can be supplied by a special apparatus (a standing calf machine) or a heavy barbell across the shoulders. Use a block under the toes and rise up as high as possible. S-T-R-E-T-C-H. Go for 20 to 30 reps with a 100-pound barbell.

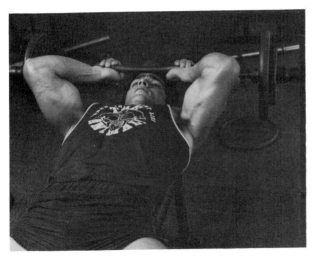 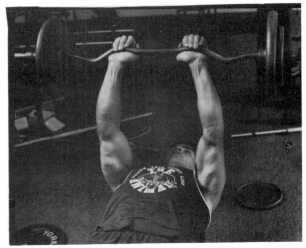

Illus. 25. Lying triceps extension (start).   *Illus. 26. Lying triceps extension (finish).*

Illus. 27. Standing calf raise (start).   *Illus. 28. Standing calf raise (finish).*

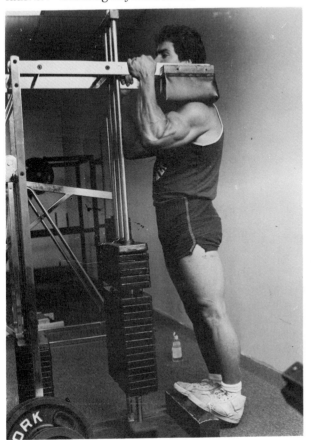 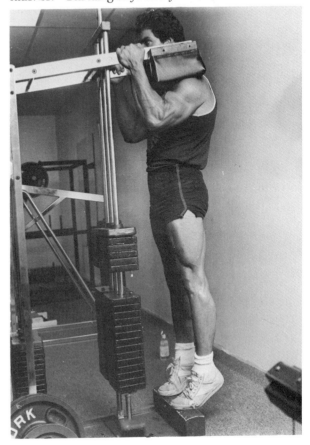

8. Crunches

Lie on the floor with your legs resting on top of an exercise bench, so that your thighs are in the vertical position. With your hands behind your head attempt to sit up. Lower and repeat. Breathe in before raising your upper body and exhale as you lower it. Crunches are good for the entire abdominal area.

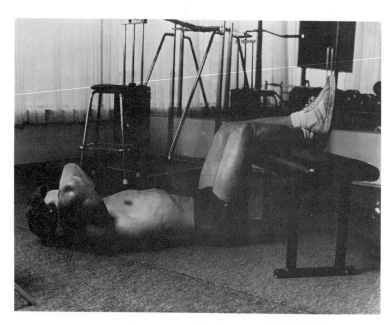

Illus. 29.   Crunches (start).

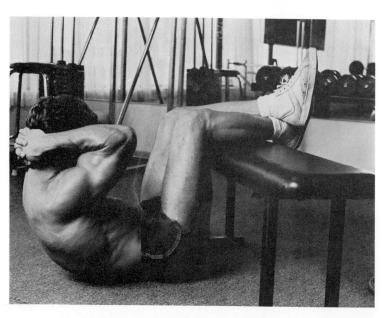

Illus. 30.   Crunches (finish).

Apparatus and Training Aids 8

Have you ever noticed the preponderance of gadgets and gizmos designed supposedly to help you become a better golfer, fisherman, or photographer?

When I was a kid I was very interested in fishing, or angling, as we called it in England. At the beginning I didn't know where to turn for advice about which type of rod or reel to purchase. Each had an endless variety of claims for why it was absolutely essential for successful fishing. I desperately wanted to be the "compleat angler" so I bought everything I could afford. Only later did I realize that 60 percent of it was totally unnecessary and half of it was outright junk.

The same happened when I took up photography: There were a million accessories to choose from. The variety of items available to today's bodybuilders is also endless.

Just what apparatus does a serious bodybuilder need to work out? Basically, a flat bench with stands and a pair of squat racks. If you cannot train with a workout partner, then both your bench and your squat racks should be fitted with a "weight safety catcher," which is a "step" or additional "cradle" into which a bar can drop if you are unable to finish a particular repetition. No one wants to be caught in the full squat position with three or four hundred pounds on his or her back, nor in the bench press supine attitude with a similar weighted bar across his or her neck!

Natural additions to your home gym after a flat bench and squat stands would be, first, an incline bench preferably "set" at about 35° (shallower than most but ideal for chest work); then a thigh extension-thigh curl machine, a chin bar, a preacher curl bench and finally you may want to allow yourself the luxury of owning a lat machine, one on which you could perform both pulldown motions and long pulley exercises and, of course, the ever-popular triceps pressdowns.

Sound like a lot? You can still do a heck of a workout with just a bench and squat stands. The other additions are not vitally important to your muscle building progress but if you can possibly afford them, they sure are nice to have around. Also nice but not necessary are hyperextension units, hack slides, calf machines, leg presses, T–bar rowing units and dip bars. I should add here that there are certain combination benches available that include virtually all the other items and accessories. If you find that you are more inclined towards these (because you are either short of funds or short of room in your home), only buy this type of combination bench *if* it is built solidly. Cheap chrome-plated, flimsy combination benches are *not* recommended.

WEIGHTS

There are two types of weights: vinyl-covered or cast-iron. Although the vinyl type are somewhat kinder to carpets, they have their drawbacks. They contain a cement filling and if repeatedly dropped or left out in the garden during the rain, they can split open and quickly become useless. Vinyl, too, is bulky and you can seldom load more than 150 pounds on a bar, often far less.

Alternatively, cast-iron weights hold far more weight per cubic foot, and can even be bought in 50- or 100-pound discs (vinyl cannot be obtained in discs weighing more than 25 pounds). Anybody serious about bodybuilding trains with disc-loading barbells, and that means iron, *never* vinyl.

Solid Weights

Some gyms are equipped with solid dumb-bells and barbells. They may be chrome plated or merely painted. To my mind these weights are definitely inferior to barbells and dumb-bells that are made up from individual discs, even though the discs may be locked in place by a welded washer.

Solid weights are *dead* weights. They can lead to injury that you might not get using disc-loaded "fixed" dumb-bells, which have a slight movement both in the handle and where the weights fit on to the bar. This small movement not only allows the hand more comfort during an exercise, but gives life and "feel" to the weight, which makes a big difference to the experienced trainer. There is also intangible pleasure in hearing the "chink" as the weight is pushed or pulled upwards, giving the serious bodybuilding enthusiast an added satisfaction as each rep is completed.

Olympic Weights

More and more bodybuilders are training with Olympic weights. In spite of the fact that Olympic weights usually cost more than double the price of regular cast iron, and that the Olympic bar will be ten times the cost of a standard bar, serious trainers never fail to seize the opportunity to hoist an Olympic bar in place of the regular cold steel. The precision engineering of the Olympic gear—the neat, knurled "correct" diameter, the perfect roll during lifting and the smoothness of action, balance and quietness of motion—makes the Olympic lifting set the Rolls Royce of exercise equipment. Not everyone can afford the luxury, but once you have used them the added training efficiency is undeniable.

Weight-Training Belt

These belts are nearly always made from thick leather, but there are synthetic weight-training belts on the market now.

Belts are necessary to the bodybuilder, especially for such exercises as squats, standing presses, rowing, cleans and deadlift movements. Their value for concentration curls, bench presses or thigh curls is dubious, although some bodybuilders insist that a belt helps *every* lift.

The main reason for wearing a belt is to add support to the lower back and there is no doubt that you can lift more in most movements wearing a belt. For example, in the squat, as your legs straighten, the tummy is inclined to push outwards, while the lower back may be under pressure to round out. A tight belt at this critical period will brace the entire midsection, hold you in to give added stability to your entire squatting action. As a consequence you will be able to use more weight, which in turn translates into more muscle.

You do not have to wear your belt for the whole workout. You can hang it up when you don't need it or simply wear it loose, tightening it just *prior* to performing the aforementioned heavy exercises. Weightlifting belts traditionally come in 4-inch and 6-inch widths. The 4-inch version is the "official" one permitted in Amateur Athletic Union competition. The 6-inch variety is not permitted in official competition because of the greater support it affords.

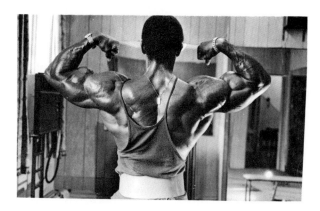

Illus. 31.   Weight-training belts are used by most bodybuilders. Model: Serge Nubret

Dipping Belts

Dipping belts are very important to the serious bodybuilder, and are worn around the hips and occasionally around the neck. Their purpose is to enable a bodybuilder to easily support additional weights while performing such exercises as dips and chins. Weight discs can be threaded on the chain part of the belt or dumb-bells hung over the chain. A dipping belt can make several nonapparatus exercises into first-class progressive resistance movements.

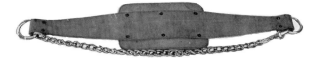

Illus. 32.   Dipping belt used for adding additional weight.

Squatting Belts

Not to be confused with the leather weight-training belt, a squatting belt is usually made from strong elasticized material and is about 12 inches wide. The idea is to offer greater midsection support, not just around the lower back, but in the entire midriff area. Tom Platz talks about bracing the torso with supports and even suggests that your sweatsuit bottoms fit the thighs tightly to give better support and overall confidence.

Squat belts, sometimes sold under the name of "health belts," are being used increasingly in gyms throughout America. They are worn in addition to the regular leather training belts.

Sweat Bands

Nothing can be more annoying than sweat trickling from your forehead into your eyes while performing an exercise such as squats, pulley work or almost any other. A sweat band not only keeps your hair away from your face, but plays an important part in preventing sweat from stinging your eyes and taking away your much-needed concentration.

Foam Pads

Foam pads are simply pieces of foam rubber that are held in the palm of your hand while training. They give the benefit of comfort and keep your hand free of calluses. They are not used widely in bodybuilding but those who do use them often swear by their efficacy. Roy Callender, Canada's undisputed best-developed man, uses foam or sponge pads in most exercises to enable him to grip the bar tightly giving complete control over the weight.

The squeezing action which is obtained when using foam pads is probably beneficial to the *quality* of your repetitions, and certainly acts to prevent slippage on the bar, which is fairly common with such exercises as wide grip bench presses and chins.

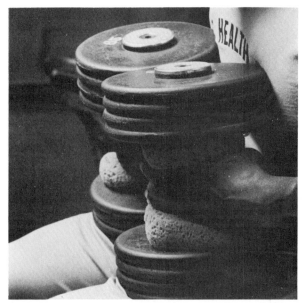

Illus. 33.   Foam or sponge pads are used to stabilize grip when training.

Gloves

Very few people wear training gloves, most preferring direct contact with the bar. Gloves serve two functions though: They prevent hands from getting severe calluses and keep sweat-ridden palms from touching the bar, which could possibly hinder your gripping power. Gloves tend to stretch and then hinder grip.

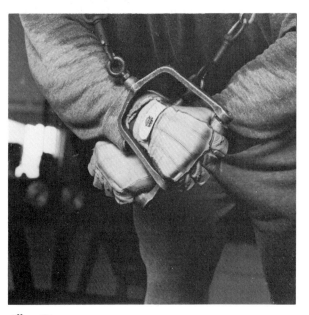

Illus. 34.

Training Straps

These aids have been around for a long time, but their popularity has been revived by heavy duty king Mike Mentzer. Training straps are usually made from strong cotton webbing and aid in lifts such as rowing, chins, shrugs, dead lifts, cleans and pulldowns where the grip is inclined to give out before the muscle being worked.

It is commonly accepted that a body can "get" several more reps of a particular exercise using training straps. And this translates into more muscle in a shorter period of time because of increased intensity in the muscle area being worked.

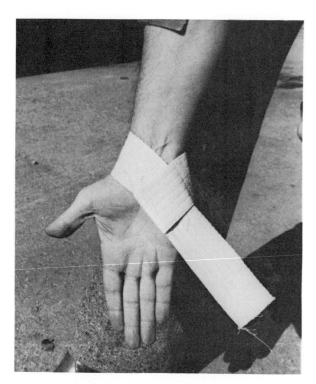

Illus. 35.   Training straps—fit around wrist.

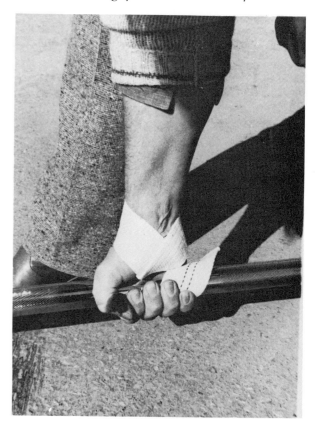

Illus. 37.   Secure grip around bar and strap.

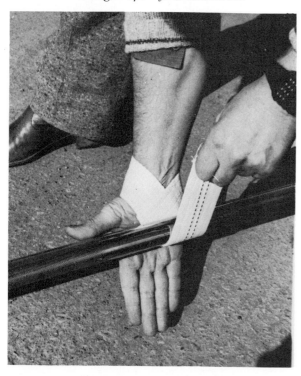

Illus. 36.   Wrap training strap around bar.

Arm Blasters

The arm blaster is a shaped aluminum strip about 5 inches wide and 24 inches long, supported at waist height by a strap around the neck. The object of the unit is to brace the elbows in an immobile state while curling barbells and dumb-bells or performing triceps pressdowns. It pretty well eliminates cheating and fosters a very strict exercise style. Arm blasters tend not to be used much by professional bodybuilders who appear to prefer working with a preacher bench to obtain the same or better effect, but it should be noted that Arnold and Franco used them extensively in their pre-Olympia training.

Illus. 38. The Joe Weider arm blaster demonstrated by Tim Belknap.

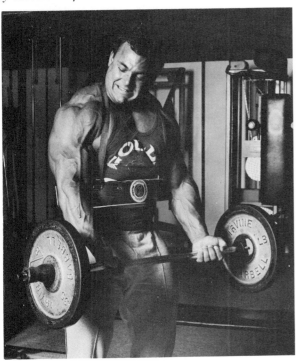

E-Z Curl Bars

If you relax your arms by your sides you will observe that the palms do not face fully to the front; they tend to face in towards the body. Cambered bars or E-Z curls were designed to allow for a more comfortable grip during exercises. The original idea was thought up to make the curling action more natural. But now some half century after their invention, E-Z curl bars are used not only for a variety of curls, including preacher bench curls and reverse curls, but they are also widely used in close-grip bench pressing and the overhead triceps stretch—with a difference. Hands are not placed on the angled hand grip areas but right at the center of the bar where the gentle curve is sufficient to hold even the sweatiest palms in place. E-Z curl bars are not superior to straight bars for curling, but they are "different" enough to bring into place alternative sets of fibres. Many established bodybuilders have found returning to the use of a straight curling bar as stimulating as their original change from straight to cambered.

Illus. 39. Mr. America Tim Belknap demonstrates the EZ curl bar.

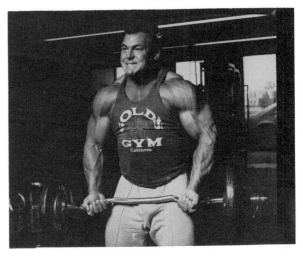

Chalk

Many bodybuilders and powerlifters and all *weightlifters* "chalk up" before attempting demanding sets. Gymnastics chalk or a bottled item brand-named *Surgrip* can be very useful to bodybuilders, especially in warm climates where the palms are prone to sweating profusely. Chalk can definitely help you hold onto that bar.

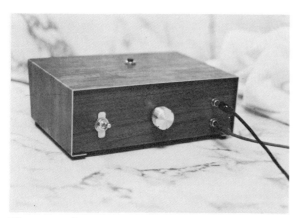

Illus. 40.   Electronic muscle stimulator.

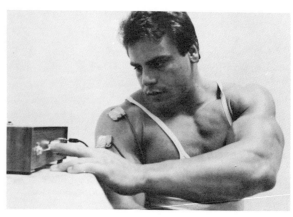

Illus. 41.   John Cardillo, one of Canada's pioneers of electronic muscle stimulators, adjusts his own machine to work the shoulder area.

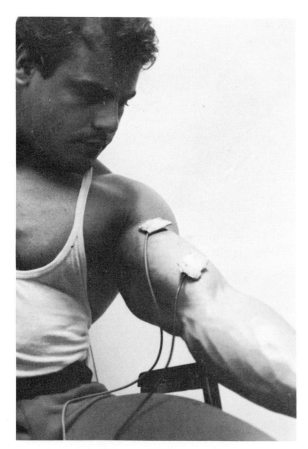

Illus. 42.   Electrodes are placed on the upper and lower parts of biceps.

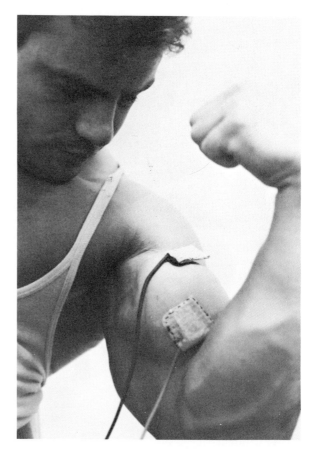

Illus. 43.   Flex arm strongly when electrodes are in place.

Electrostimulators

Electrical stimulation machines have been around for over 20 years. You may have even used one in your high school science class to get a reflex in a dead frog's leg.

Electrical stimulation is a proven aid to strengthening, rehabilitating and actually building muscles. In fact Dr. Charles Godfrey, head of the rehabilitation department at Toronto's Wellesley Hospital, made a formal study which concluded that "there is greater average improvement with electrostimulation than with exercise, and it's faster and easier."

Both bodybuilders and weightlifters have used stimulators with good results. Mike Mentzer has used them extensively. Canadian bodybuilder John Cardillo, an authority on these machines, has often used them in his training.

Basically, tetanizing muscle stimulation involves applying two electrode pads (which are dampened with a wet cloth first) near either end of the muscle, and conducting a current through it until the muscle contracts and knots up into a cramp. All skeletal muscles are compatible with electric stimulator machines. The heart is not.

Mild electrostimulation is of very little value. As in weight training, the muscles must be fully loaded on a progressive basis. Underloading a muscle, minimal exercise, is useless. Loading the muscle to full capacity leads to maximum strength.

There could possibly be a degree of danger if excessive stimulation is used on a muscle in that you could sustain a tear or strain. Accordingly, these machines are usually only available through a doctor's, chiropractor's or physiotherapist's direct recommendation or prescription.

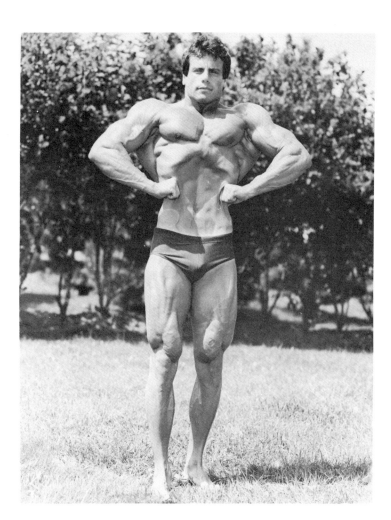

Illus. 44.   John Cardillo: Canada's pioneer of electronic stimulator bodybuilding.

Inversion Boots

Originally known as "anti-gravity boots," these are specially designed lightweight "shoes" which fit around the ankle and enable a person to hang safely upside down from a horizontal bar.

Inversion boots are surprisingly comfortable and easy to use. They definitely help stretch the spine and back which gives relief to certain forms of back problems.

Although inversion boots have been used by champions like Frank Zane, Vince Gironda, Brad Harris, Frank Calta and Franco Columbu, they are not considered a necessary part of the hardcore bodybuilder's artillery.

Over 40 years ago, John Grimek performed numerous upside-down exercises using homemade leg straps and would exercise with rows, curls and even inverted squats using dumb-bells.

Today bodybuilders perform a variety of exercises with and without weights using inversion boots, but these are still only beneficial in adding variety to one's training. In my opinion the single most effective exercise using inversion boots is the upside-down sit-up. This movement vigorously works that all-important lower abdomen down near the groin. Few exercises work this important area as effectively.

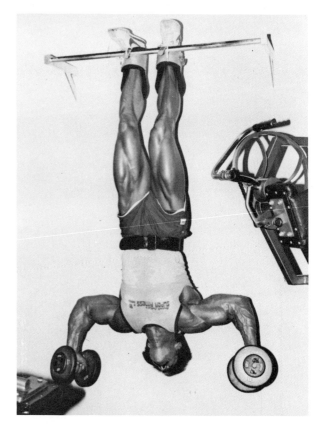

Illus. 45. Frank Calta demonstrates Inversion Boots, bodybuilding's newest training aid.

Just about everybody knows that free weight training and the use of related weight-loaded apparatus are the best ways to build strength and muscle. But how many advertisements would have you believe otherwise?

The market has been flooded during the last hundred years with items claiming to build muscles faster than with conventional weight training. Some even claim to build your body in "just 60 seconds a day."

The large variety of small exercise apparatus, some better than others admittedly, are all positively second-rate compared to the results obtainable from the use of free weight training.

Some mail-order courses like *Universal Bodybuilding, Weider's Mr. America Course, Olympic Musclebuilders* and *Muscle Fighter IV* offer a combined nonapparatus *and* apparatus program. A beginner could start by performing nonapparatus exercises and then graduate to the more advanced weight training movements. In fact, many top bodybuilders do perform certain nonapparatus exercises in their workouts.

Different types of floor dips are commonly used as are all types of chins and parallel bar dips (both of which are termed nonapparatus since they do not involve barbells or dumb-bells). The point against nonapparatus training (one not agreed upon by the Atlas Company) is that you cannot build your body to its maximum potential using nonapparatus training exclusively. Nonapparatus training does not allow unlimited progressive resistance to be applied to every movement as regular weight training allows merely by adding a weight disc to the bar when your strength increases.

When you have doubts or reservations about something in this sport, try to think it out for yourself. If it sounds bigger than life, or almost impossible, chances are it is!

Dynamic Diet and Super Supplementation 9

Bodybuilders know that muscle size is stimulated by regularly performed high-intensity workouts. They also know that, once stimulated into growth, muscles depend solely on diet to build or reduce their weight: the type and quantity of food are of great importance.

Nutrition could be compared to a bank account. By substituting calories (units of heat; energy) for dollars, you start with a given amount of money in the bank. Eating is like making deposits, in that you add to the total in the bank. Writing a check can be regarded as exercise (walking, breathing, weight training, running) and subtracted from the amount in the account. If your deposits equal your withdrawals, your balance (weight) will stay the same. If you spend as many calories as you eat, your body will stay the same. Burn more calories than you consume and your body will start losing weight (muscle and fat). In practice, for example, if you eliminate just one pat of butter a day, you will not deposit some 3,780 calories each month! This represents one pound of body weight (and 12 pounds a year). Eliminate two pats of butter per day and you're losing about half a pound a week.

Just as you have to pay into your bank account in genuine currency to accrue the long-term benefits, so do you have to eat genuine food to build up a healthy, dynamic physique. Synthetic foods may seem to be o.k. when first deposited, but like the bounced check, their value is temporary, and if you continue to ingest them, you will soon become physically bankrupt.

This is not to say that everything that passes your lips must be 100 percent perfect nutrition, but it sure helps if the majority of what you eat is good, wholesome food.

So what *is* good nutrition? Opinions vary as to exactly how much of what kinds of food we require for a balanced eating program. Generally one should select from the five main food groups:

1. Milk group—Milk, cheese, yoghurt

2. Meat group—Beef, lamb, pork, poultry, eggs, fish, veal;

3. Vegetable/Fruit group

4. Bread/Grain group

5. Fats/Oil group—Butter, margarine, salad oil (usually only small amounts of these).

This is not a book for the health faddist, but for the hardcore bodybuilder, whose main desire is learning how to eat to get big fast.

We need to eat well to build a power-packed body. Forget any substandard diet that barely allows you to pass from one day to another with minimal bodybuilding gains. You train hard for your muscles. Don't let your effort be wasted by ignoring the importance of optimum nourishment. Go for only the best!

To understand exactly what constitutes the best we should first consider the worst. Never mind the "experts" who tell you that batter-dipped fish and

Approximate Nutrient Value of Fast-Food

Based on data from *Dietetic Currents* (Vol. 5, 1978) and
Nutrient Value of Some Common Foods (Health & Welfare, Canada, Rev. 1979)

	Calories	Fat	Protein	Carbo-hydrates	Calcium	Iron	Magne-sium	Salt (Sodium)	Vitamin A	Vitamin (B-Complex)	Vitamin C	Fibre
Recommended daily nutrient intake (RDNI)	2,100	35% of calories or less	41 g.	50–55% of calories	700 mg.	14 mg.	250 mg.	2,000–3,000 mg. a day suggested	800 RE	Differs for each B vitamin	30 mg.	Not officially specified
Meal 1 (Hamburger)	1,200	50 g. or about 38% of calories in the meal	30 g.	140 g. or about 47% of calories	430 mg.	4.4 mg.	90 mg.	1,400 mg.	Low	Adequate (except B_6)	22 mg.	Low
Meal 2 (Pizza and salad—levels depend on salad items)	980	26 g. or about 24% of calories	29 g.	120 g. or about 49% of calories	500 mg.	5 mg.	28 mg.	1,800 mg.	Fair	Fair	27 mg.	Adequate
Meal 3 (Chicken)	1,490	70 g. or about 42% of calories	62 g.	140 g. or about 38% of calories	200 mg.	4.5 mg.	30 mg.	2,290 mg.	Low	Adequate	27 mg.	Fair
Meal 4 (Hot dog)	810	25 g. or about 28% of calories	15 g.	55 g. or about 27% of calories	100 mg.	3 mg.	30 mg.	1,300 mg.	Low	Low	12 mg.	Low
Meal 5 (Fish & chips)	1,350	60 g. or about 40% of calories	28 g.	130 g. or about 39% of calories	420 mg.	4.5 mg.	100 mg.	1,700 mg.	Sufficient	Ample (except B_6)	18 mg. 18 mg.	Fair Fair

chips constitute a well-balanced meal, that a Big Mac® is the highest quality fast-food in the world, or that pizza is nutritionally balanced. Forget it! Fast-food has become a part of our diet, but let's keep it to as few visits as possible. You are not going to acquire a prize-winning body chomping down hot dogs and pizzas, hamburgers and spaghetti, most of which have high salt (sodium) and only fair-to-low fibre content.

As for thirst quenchers like sodas and other carbonated soft drinks, chances are you'd get more nutrition if you popped a sugar cube in a glass of brown dye and topped it up with rainwater. Come to think of it, the cola companies buy more brown dye than all other industries on earth combined!

The products that you should eat only occasionally because they are either nutritionally bankrupt or full of sodium, sugar, chemicals, preservatives, coloring dyes or artificial flavors include: synthetic or packaged cakes, pies, cookies, "creams" (if it's spelled kreme, creem, kreem, kream, creme, creame or kreame, it ain't real), doughnuts, puddings, candies, spaghetti, pizza, hot dogs, smoked meats, potato chips, chocolate bars, beer, pretzels, ice cream and ices, jam, soft drinks, salad dressings, dyed meats, bacon, packaged ham, synthetic sausages, sugary breakfast cereals and other "junk" foods. In decaffeinated coffee, caffeine is removed from coffee beans with methylenechloride, a chemical solvent suspected of causing cancer. Steer away from regular consumption of white flour products, sugar-loaded canned fruits and vegetables, gravies and deep fried foods of all kinds.

By now you may be wondering just what you *can* eat! The answer of course is to keep to natural foods as much as possible. We've listed the worst—now for the best.

Make up your meals from wholesome unspoiled foods such as 100 percent wheat bread (if it has "whole wheat" or "whole rye" on it, it's good). Natural "complex" carbohydrate foods are best. Base your diet on fresh, broiled meats and poultry, fish, eggs, unsalted nuts, fruits and fresh vegetables and salads. Steam your vegetables; do not boil them. Never fry meat or fish. Don't remove the peel from apples, tomatoes, peaches and so on: It contains nutrients that the fruit itself does not. Be sure to wash your fruits and vegetables thoroughly since they may have been sprayed with harmful pesticides or insecticides.

Often bodybuilders will ask me about which foods are the very best, the superfoods! "What can I

eat for fantastic energy and stamina? For huge muscle size, definition and separation?" My answer disappoints them: There are *no* miracle foods. There is no such thing as a super-diet that will make your body functions better than normal, because food is not magic and normal is the best you can get. There's a heck of a lot of bad food around that given time can turn you into a physical and mental wreck, but there is no secret food that will work better than *normal, wholesome foods.*

When you are eating the best natural, wholesome foods, you are doing everything possible to reach perfection, nutritionally. If you eat a meal which, for example, consists of real orange juice, fresh salad, baked free-ranging poultry, jacketed potato, lightly steamed vegetables and fresh fruit salad, you deserve a perfect ten. On the other hand, start the meal with a beer, follow with deep-fried batter-coated chicken, french fries, canned sugar-loaded vegetables, mopping up the salty gravy with devitalized white bread (suitably treated with chemicals to lengthen its shelf life and to give the appearance of freshness) and concluding with ice cream, canned fruit and after-dinner mints, and I will give you a "zero" plus a dose of bicarbonate of soda and the address of the nearest specialist in arthritis and degenerative disease!

Here are samples of good bodybuilding diets which give you a guideline for success:
Breakfast
1. Citrus fruit or fruit juices such as orange, grapefruit, lime, lemon, tomato
2. Whole grain cereal with milk and fresh fruit
3. Two boiled eggs or boiled fish or sliced lean ham
4. Whole wheat or rye toast and honey
5. Glass of milk or fresh weak tea or decaffeinated coffee
Lunch
1. Homemade vegetable or meat broth
2. Rye or wheat bread cheese sandwich, or sliced meat and salad or natural yoghurt and fresh fruit
Dinner
1. Salad, soup, grapefruit, shrimp cocktail or fresh fruit juice
2. Eight oz. broiled steak, veal chop, liver, chicken or salmon steak, etc.
3. Steamed broccoli, cauliflower, carrots or spinach, etc.
4. Fresh melon, yoghurt or mixed fruit salad

You better believe you are what you eat. Go for the best foods and you will feel like a million bucks. Combine positive eating with really motivated training and you will look like a million too!

I often get asked which is the best weight-gaining food. As mentioned earlier, the answer is probably milk. All young mammals increase, double, triple their body weight as a result of drinking milk from day one. It is the almost perfect food, containing virtually all the essential nutrients discovered by man, in correct proportions. It undoubtedly even contains the undiscovered vitamins and essential ingredients.

As a bodybuilding food you should take your milk as an extra, not as a meal in itself. Take it between meals, not, however, just before a meal because it could interfere with your appetite. It doesn't much matter which type of milk you take, whole (homogenized), low-fat or skimmed . . . the goodness is still there and your muscles will get nourishment. Some adults, however, lack the enzyme lactase to digest the sugar in milk. They should try a new product Lactaid® that helps *their* system break down lactose (milk sugar), or try it in small amounts with meals.

Never miss breakfast. It may be the hardest meal to stomach, but to the bodybuilder it is absolutely essential. When bodybuilders complain that they can't make progress, one of the first questions I ask them is: "What do you eat for breakfast?" Quite often the reply comes back: "Oh! I don't eat any breakfast, I don't have time."

Most people eat at night around six or seven o'clock. The next meal, breakfast, doesn't come until seven or eight the next morning, over twelve hours away. If you miss breakfast, your stomach will go without food for a full sixteen or more hours—too long. It's crazy even for a person trying to lose weight to miss breakfast; for the bodybuilder it is sheer lunacy.

The best, although not necessarily the only, way to eat your food is to take five or six small meals throughout the day instead of the traditional two or three larger ones. Heavy meals tend to sap one's energy and actually can be too much stress on the system for comfort; better that your body be fed more frequently, in smaller quantitites. After all, the body can utilize only a certain amount at one time (anything over 25 grams of protein in one sitting, for example, is a waste). Smaller meals are more easily digested and maintain a constant source of energy and nutriment to the bodybuilder. In short, you will make better bodybuilding gains. By all means keep to your traditional breakfast, lunch and supper, but do not stuff yourself. Never gobble huge platefuls of potatoes, rice or meat with gravy until it hurts. Ideal snacks to take between lunch and supper, breakfast and lunch or mid-evening include cheese sandwiches, small omelettes, yoghurt and fruit, shredded wheat and milk or peanut butter sandwiches.

There is a large variance in the amounts of protein we require, depending on a variety of factors including health, age, sex, size and training habits. Actually the larger and younger you are, the more you need. To estimate your own personal daily recommended allowance, see the chart below:

AGE	POUND KEY
11–14	0.45
15–18	0.40
19 and over	0.36

Find the pound key under your age group. Multiply that figure by your weight. The result will be your daily protein requirement in grams.

For example, if you are 29 years old and weigh 150 pounds, your pound key is 0.36; $150 \times 0.36 = 54$ g., your daily protein requirement.

Most people need at least 45 grams of protein daily. Naturally if you are keen to build up solid weight, it is always good to bear in mind that it is better to be *over* your minimum daily requirement than *under*. If you take in less protein than you require, your body will rob your muscles to make sure that it gets enough protein to keep essential mechanisms such as your heart and lungs working efficiently. Remove the water from your muscles and what you have left is practically *all* protein. If the body has to rob your muscles of protein to function, they will get smaller.

On the other hand, if you regularly take in large amounts of protein well in excess of your requirements, it will not adorn your frame as pure muscle—it will go on as fat! A gram of protein has the same amount of calories as a gram of carbohydrate—four. (A gram of fat has nine and a gram of alcohol yields 7 calories—or 198 calories per ounce.)

There are basically two types of protein—complete and incomplete.

Complete protein, found mainly in foods of animal origin such as meats, poultry, seafood, eggs, milk and cheese, provides the proper balance of nine essential amino acids that build tissues. Of late, spirulina, a freshwater algae, has also been discovered to be a complete protein.

Incomplete protein such as is found in seeds, nuts, peas, grains and beans lacks certain essential amino acids and is not used efficiently when eaten alone. When it is combined with even small amounts of animal-source protein, however, it becomes complete.

The universal question in bodybuilding is "How do I get bigger as fast as possible—*without* getting fat. I just want to build a huge amount of muscle size!" Well, don't we all!

Are supplements necessary? Do they help the physique grow faster? The easy gainer doesn't need them, but most beginning bodybuilders use supplements to help gain size. When Arnold Schwarzenegger first came to California, he would, after a workout, down a huge container of milk and egg protein mixed with a couple of quarts of milk. Ironically, later in his career he found he could regain his muscle mass without the use of supplements. Maybe muscle memory has something to do with it; they say it's easy to get 20-inch arms the second time around.

For anyone who isn't able to get his or her daily protein requirements from regular meals, whole food protein supplements are helpful. The best formulas are either an egg, meat, seafood or milk protein, or a combination. Very common mixtures are egg and milk or soya and milk. A milk or milk and egg protein powder supplement offers all the essential amino acids and can be completely utilized. On the other hand, a soya-based protein powder may not be fully usable, unless mixed with high protein from an animal source such as milk.

Protein supplements come in liquid or powder form and are available in health food stores with or without carbohydrates or fats. They generally supply about 24 grams of protein per ounce (two heaping tablespoons), about the equivalent protein value of a three-ounce steak.

Do not make the mistake of thinking that protein is nonfattening. Any food that has significant calorie content is potentially fattening.

These rules of thumb can guide you in calorieland:

Leave the table hungry and you will lose weight.

Leave the table satisfied and you will maintain weight.

Leave the table full and you will gain weight.

Muscles are made of protein so it stands to reason that a muscle that is worked by heavy weights, and on which a demand has been placed to get bigger, should be fed sufficient protein. And what better way to do it than to take protein supplementation in the form of a pleasant-tasting shake?

Most protein supplements mix a protein powder (milk and egg is the most popular) with either a juice or plain milk. You may of course add all types of flavoring, such as chocolate, strawberries, bananas, etc.

The best time to take your protein shake is between supper and going to bed, about 9:30 at night. It will act as a protein snack and feed the muscles while you sleep. If you are trying to gain muscular body weight, do not take a protein supplement in place of a meal. Take it as an *extra*. You may take a protein supplement more than once a day, but since the body can only assimilate about 20 to 25 grams of protein at any one time, you will be paying out your hard-earned dollars for the dubious honor of having the most protein-rich urine in town.

Many bodybuilders lay great importance on what have become known as "glandulars," touted in recent years as the natural substitute for steroids. Actually glandulars are nothing new. Bodybuilders have been taking desiccated liver tablets for years. Nutrition expert Vince Gironda has recommended taking several liver tablets every hour during the day to keep a high protein supply in the blood stream. Many hard-training bodybuilders have found this works!

As for other glandulars such as pancreas, kidney, heart, adrenal and pituitary, it would seem that they contain a variety of very high-quality nutrients like their whole food counterparts and, accordingly, would prove especially effective for those who were not already getting adequate, balanced nutrition. The claim that glandulars would give the same muscle-building effect as steroids is doubtful.

It is my belief that every bodybuilder should take a one-a-day vitamin mineral pill daily with a meal to assure adequate daily nutrition. It costs pennies a day and there is no chance of upsetting your system with toxicity since the dosages in such pills are always minimal.

There are several supplements that bodybuilders take in the belief that they help remove fat from the body. Whether this is true or not is a moot point. Certainly there are no *miraculous* foods which cause the body to burn up fat. But, in conjunction with a low-calorie diet, these substances may help to *slightly* decrease body fat.

Choline

Usually taken with inositol, choline is a member of the B-complex family of vitamins and is a lipotropic (fat emulsifier). It works with inositol (another B-complex vitamin) to utilize fats and cholesterol.

To my knowledge the first champion bodybuilders to use choline and inositol were Larry Scott and Zabo Kozewski back in the 1960s. The recommended daily allowance has not yet been established, but it is estimated that the average adult diet contains between 500 and 900 mg. a day. Evidence at present appears to show that choline emulsifies cholesterol so it doesn't settle on artery walls or in the gall bladder. There is also evidence that choline can help to ameliorate the problem of memory loss in later years and to eliminate poisons and drugs from your system by aiding the liver.

The usual supplement dosage is 500 to 1,000 mg. daily and there is no known toxicity, which means it is unlikely that taking too much would upset your system.

Inositol

Inositol is best taken together with choline. (The two together form lecithin.) Like choline, it has been found important in nourishing brain cells and also promotes healthy hair and prevents eczema. It is debatable whether inositol and choline affect the fat content of your body to the extent of improving definition. Many bodybuilders believe that when choline and inositol are taken prior to a contest in conjunction with the usual low calorie pre-competition diet, there is a positive effect. The skin, they say, does get thinner, and the muscles show up more.

Kelp

Twenty years ago, kelp was believed to help speed up a slow or even a normal metabolism. Bodybuilders in need of more definition believed that taking large amounts of kelp would increase the fat-burning process. This is not now generally believed to be true. Kelp is not even the super source of minerals once believed, and it does contain undesirably high amounts of sodium (salt) which promotes water retention, the last thing a competing bodybuilder needs.

Dr. Michael Walczak, the bodybuilders' doctor, and one of the most knowledgeable men on the subject of nutrition for weight trainers, states in his excellent book, *Nutrition and Wellbeing:* "The practice of using kelp (iodine) in the role of activating thyroid metabolic function is a fallacy."

Thyomucase®

This is a relatively new drug which can be injected or rubbed on the skin surface as a cream. It apparently originated in France and is made from the urine of pregnant women. Its purpose is to remove fat from just under the skin, and whether it works or not is still debatable. If it does work, it only does so in conjunction with a reduced-calorie diet. The fad for taking thyomucase appears to be waning. Some bodybuilders have experienced acute burns from using the "thyo" creams.

Drugs–
The Illusory "Edge" 10

"It appears that anabolic steroids can accelerate the acquisition of muscular strength and power and simultaneously permit training at or near maximum capacity with greater frequency."

That quote from Dr. John P. O'Shea of Oregon University was published by the American Association for the Advancement of Science some twenty years ago, and along with thousands of other pro-steroid quotations, is at least partly responsible for the state many of our bodybuilders are in today.

Artificial steroids do aid in muscle growth and strength, especially in those who train hard and ingest plenty of protein foods. There is just one little catch. They will put you on a dialysis machine faster than it takes you to win the Mr. Novice, let alone the Mr. America, title. A dialysis machine does the work of malfunctioning kidneys. The treatment can last all day and one has to have the treatment twice a week—for life.

Artificial anabolic steroids were invented in 1938. They were produced to aid war victims, fire casualties and the aged (especially after illness or operations) to gain strength and weight. The fact that steroids had undesirable side effects didn't seem to matter at that time because they were being administered to those already hanging onto life by a thread.

The IFBB (International Federation of Bodybuilders) does not endorse doping or the taking of artificial growth hormones (androgens).

Nor does the International Olympic Committee (IOC). In May, 1967, their medical committee reported to the IOC's 67th Session in Teheran:

"The IOC considers that the use of anabolic steroids (except for medical purposes) constitutes *doping* from the Olympic viewpoint." Subsequently the IOC banned steroid use and introduced stringent steroid tests.

Today in Britain, Canada and the U.S.A. a few bodybuilding shows include steroid tests. These are called *natural* bodybuilding contests because all who take part are free from artificial anabolic steroids. Surely they are the wave of the future. But the problem exists on a huge scale. Not only do professional bodybuilders take steroids to help them win contests, but even school kids and novice bodybuilders take them . . . and take them . . . and take them. Fellows who do not have a prayer of winning contests because of some genetic flaw ingest steroids until their vital organs are ruined beyond repair.

Virtually every city in North America has a gym which distributes anabolic steroids. Often the gym owner has a drawer full of hypodermic needles, and will refer to the treatment as "your B_{12} shots."

Of course in some cases a gym member may legitimately be getting B$_{12}$ shots, but more often than you'd expect, the substance is artificial anabolic steroid. The gym owner may attempt to cover himself by having a local doctor write the prescription and even administer the drug. But where in the Hippocratic oath does a doctor get the right to administer drugs to sportsmen in perfect health?

If a gym owner ever offers you artificial steroids, go to your local medical association and register an official complaint. Tell the Better Business Bureau about him, and make the gym owner pay back your entire fee. Then go to the local chamber of commerce and make them act against the offender. The sooner he is put out of commission the better. Too many innocent youngsters have been taken advantage of this way: While they suffer the problems caused by the drugs, the creeps who sell them are laughing all the way to the bank.

According to national bodybuilding champion Rod Koontz, some misguided bodybuilders who take steroids to gain weight are also taking thyroid to cut up (get definition), speed to train hard, weed to come back down to get some sleep, Ritalin® to make it easier to diet, Thyomucase® to thin the skin, and Quaaludes® so they don't feel the pain of training.

Misguided they most definitely are, because these drugs will sooner or later knock out even the ruggedest bodybuilder. Steroids are hormones. They contribute to a constructive metabolic process that turns food into living tissue. They can also be hepatic (affect one's liver); carcinogenic (contribute to cancer); responsible for "undue edema" (give one dropsy), and can promote coronary thrombosis (heart attack).

In his book *Anabolic Steroids and Sports* (Sports Science Consultants, Natick, Massachusetts, 1978), Dr. James E. Wright, without condoning the use of steroids, tries to get laymen to understand why an athlete may take steroids. He quotes a world-class athlete whom he interviewed:

"Think about how small the differences usually are between first and second place, between winning and losing (in high level competition). And keep in mind the drive and ambition and the competitive spirit of somebody competing at that level. Think about the time, the energy, and the pain invested . . . The financial rewards are, in most cases, minimal . . . I hate to admit it, but an obsessive-compulsive personality is practically a requirement (for success at these levels). . . . The advice I value most is from people who've been there. . . . The average guy on the street, and even lots of people in sports obviously don't understand the pressures. . . . It's like everything else in life: when it all gets down to the nitty-gritty, you grab anything you can that might give you a winning edge."

It is true, however, that bodybuilders do not like taking steroids. But because their competition is taking them and gaining an edge, they believe that they too must join the pack or be left behind. One top professional bodybuilder who wished to remain anonymous told me: "There are twenty-five different types of anabolic steroids in existence today and some are safer to take than others.

"I usually benefit from taking steroids while training for a top pro contest, I find I gain the most benefit from these drugs when I'm dieting very hard. The main advantage for me is that they retain the size in the muscles while I'm burning away body fat. But, of course, I have to have the correct amount of protein balance in my body or the steroids will not work."

Curiously, because most bodybuilders shave their bodies before a competition or a photo session, the uninitiated layman, sensing something "abnormal" (a plucked turkey appearance?), has often accused the bodybuilder of having "synthetic-looking" muscles.

With the wide use of steroids, the bodybuilder at last gives weight to the layman's original argument which for years had no truth, but now alas, stings with the sorry reality that at least a percentage of most top bodybuilders' muscles is the result of a pill or a hypodermic needle.

The strong movement to rid bodybuilding and other sports of anabolic steroids gained impetus when the International Federation of Bodybuilders, as a service to the International Sports Federation, presented a report based on research conducted by James E. Wright, Ph.D. entitled "Anabolic-Androgenic Steroids in Sport." The report dealt in depth with the entire question, especially from the bodybuilders' point of view, and resoundingly concluded that no title or sports achievement is worth risking one's mental and physical health.

IFBB head Ben Weider also has personally known individuals who have seriously harmed their health and physique as the result of heavy steroid consumption. In a couple of cases the fellows were teenagers who cried when their doctors related the seriousness of the damage and, too late, they wondered why they had been so incredibly stupid!

Thyomucase is another drug that has been used

extensively by bodybuilders to reduce fat levels. It was first brought over to this country from France by Serge Nubret whose sister is a pharmacist. It can apparently be bought over the counter without a doctor's prescription. According to Dr. Michael Walczak, the bodybuilders' doctor: "Thyomucase is a mucopolysaccharide extracted from testicular tissue. Its function is to remove premenstrual edema from the female body. In France, thyomucase is used in combination with a 500-calorie-a-day diet to combat cellulite. It's available in injectable form, as a cream and as a suppository.

Thyomucase should not be confused with hylaluronidase, which is marketed in North America under the name Wydase®. Many bodybuilders have become extremely sick using this product. This is documented by Dr. Walczak: "hylaluronidase is an active enzyme, with many undesirable side effects. It is an extremely dangerous drug when used to achieve muscular definition and it actually does nothing to help a bodybuilder cut up for a show. Hylaluronidase is believed to be the destructive agent in spider and snake venom, and actually tends to cause body bloat rather than loss of water under the skin."

The thyroid gland is the control monitor responsible for regulating metabolism. The basal metabolic rate is the rate at which your body burns up fuel at rest. It can be likened to the "tick-over" or idle rate of a car. Whereas some people have a very active thyroid, and accordingly are highly strung, overactive and have fast metabolisms, others have comparatively slow metabolism, possibly caused by an underactive thyroid.

In order to capitalize on this, some bodybuilders in need of a super-defined (low-fat) physique at contest time have taken to using thyroxin to stimulate additional thyroid activity, even though their own thyroid glands may be entirely normal, to speed the metabolic process. Starting with one grain, they build to two, three and more grains as the contest approaches. This is an extremely unwise practice. For one thing, your own thyroid gland, no longer producing its own thyroxin, may shut off entirely. After the contest, when a bodybuilder ceases to take thyroxin, he could bloat up enormously, his body taking on a feminine appearance, because his natural supply of thyroxin has ceased. It is no exaggeration to say that shortsighted bodybuilders who have taken "therapeutic" doses of steroids and other chemicals have permanently damaged their health, and in numerous cases, have brought about untimely death.

As much as anyone I appreciate the pressing need of the aspiring bodybuilder for fast muscular development. He wants the ultimate in size and muscularity, and will do almost anything to attain his goal. My advice is: Do almost anything, but stop short of the total lunacy of drug abuse.

Shoulders 11

Wide shoulders have been a symbol of masculinity ever since the beginning of human existence. Your actual width is pretty well determined by your clavical length: The "stretch" of your collarbones (biacromial) limits the degree of impressiveness. Of course your shoulders will look more formidable by adding muscle tissue and if you already have wide bones, they will look even better when you add muscle.

The question as to whether a man can widen his shoulders through exercise or any other means has long been discussed. The consensus is that after the age of 25 or so, it is virtually impossible to widen the biacromial width. Prior to that age the clavicles grow fractionally in length when regular support stress is placed on them in heavy exercise such as hand balancing, gymnastics or progressive weight training. Some thickening of these bones under these stresses will occur.

The best exercises for aiding the bone-widening process include heavy presses of all kinds and straight-arm pullovers. Bear in mind, however, that a small amount of exercise over a limited time period will not effect much growth. In fact, even large amounts of heavy exercise over a limited period will not effect much growth. And even large amounts of heavy exercise over a period of several years will only widen the bone width slightly. This is not a process which sees extravagant gains. Your results will be concomitant with your efforts, but even the most determined trainers will only gain a small reward in actual bony shoulder width.

Deltoid muscle development, actual shoulder growth, is another thing entirely. Big melon-like deltoids can be yours. And even if you have naturally narrow shoulders they can become darned impressive by adding plenty of muscle size to all three deltoid heads. The deltoid, like the triceps of the upper arm, is a three-headed muscle and it is advisable to build all three heads for full, rounded development.

Twenty years ago this did not matter. A bodybuilder would seldom deliberately work his back or front deltoids, concentrate instead on building the side (lateral) head to add more width. Things are different today. Bodybuilding has come of age and contest judges are more discriminating. If a contestant is lacking in side, front or rear deltoid development he will be penalized accordingly.

Here are the reasons why you need to develop all three deltoid areas:

Side (Lateral) Deltoid

This is the part of your shoulders that actually adds width. Pack muscle bulk onto your sides, just an inch on either side and you will completely change your appearance. If you doubt me, try this simple test. Slip into a tight sweat or tee shirt and place a rolled up sock or handkerchief underneath the sweater on the outer sides of each shoulders. Now take a look in the mirror. Just an inch more width either side and you look like Hercules unchained.

Rear (Posterior) Deltoid

Development of the back of your shoulders is a must. It greatly improves your posterior appearance, preventing you from looking round-shouldered. It also gives your shoulder thickness from the side, and when viewed relaxed from the rear, well-developed posterior deltoids add that important detail to overall back impressiveness.

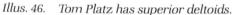

Illus. 46.   Tom Platz has superior deltoids.

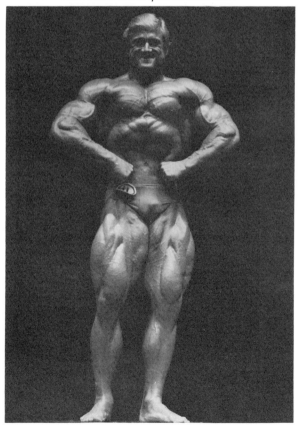

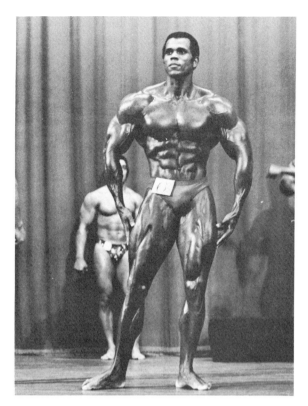

Illus. 47.   One of the greatest—Serge Nubret shows how wide shoulders complement the physique.

Front (Anterior) Deltoid

It used to be fashionable to "tie in" the front deltoids with the upper pecs. This was accomplished with plenty of incline barbell presses and facilitated by the fact that bodybuilders had higher percentages of fat in former days.

Today, pec tie-ins are out. Rather than trying to develop pecs that flow into the delts, today's bodybuilders build the pecs as one muscle, and work the front deltoid as a separate area. This separation actually aids the upper body appearance and, contrary to popular opinion, a bulging front deltoid helps your "visual" width because any form of cross lighting will show it up as a separate entity and the ultimate effect is broader shoulders.

Most people enjoy working the shoulders. There are a variety of pushing and pulling motions that exercise the delts and the shoulders respond well in most cases. They get a good pump and growth is normally fairly rapid.

All forms of pressing movements, while in the upright position, strenuously work the shoulders. Olympic lifters involved in pressing and jerking heavy weights overhead invariably have large, well rounded shoulders.

It is often a good idea to start off your shoulder routine with several sets of heavy (quality) shoulder work, such as the press-behind-neck exercise, and conclude the routine with isolation exercises such as lateral raises, front raises, etc. Of course the pre-exhaust method contradicts this situation (see chapter 23 on pre-exhaust), but it is the variety and "shockability" of your routines that keep the muscles growing. A complete reversal of procedure often stimulates additional growth.

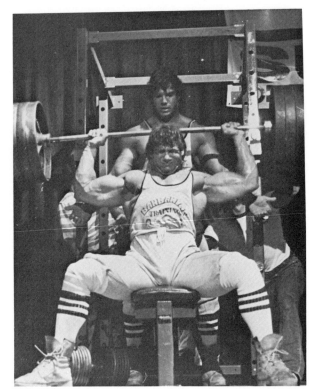

Illus. 49.   Barbarian Peter Paul shows the start of a mammoth press behind neck.

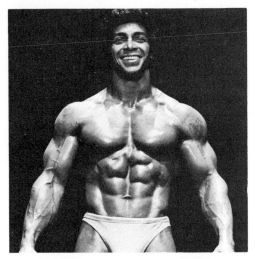

Illus. 48.   Harold Poole (USA) has full wide shoulders.

Press Behind Neck (from Racks)

Although it is not absolutely necessary, you will find that you get better results by placing the loaded barbell on squat racks prior to doing the press behind neck. This eliminates the energy-consuming cleaning of the weight (bringing it from floor to shoulder) plus the wasted motion of getting it into position behind your neck.

Duck under the bar, with your hands set about 28 to 32 inches apart. Press upwards while standing or sitting erect, being careful to hold your elbows back throughout the movement. As soon as the arms straighten, return and repeat. Some people prefer to lock out (lock the elbows as arms straighten) each rep while others feel this is unnecessary. Both styles work and whether or not you choose to lock out is up to you. After the set, return the barbell to the racks.

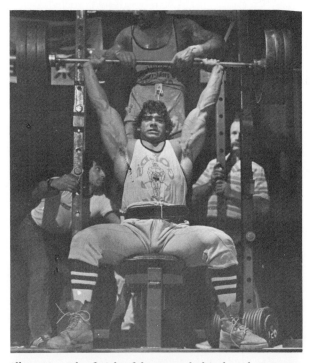

Illus. 50.   The finish of the press behind neck. Peter does 315 lbs for 10 reps. Incredible!

Upright Row

To properly work the shoulder muscles and not the trapezius, you should grasp the barbell with hands a shoulder width apart.

Raise and lower the bar, palms facing down, elbows held as high as possible throughout the exercise. Keep the action rhythmic. You may hold the barbell out away from the body during this exercise if you wish. It puts a little more "constant" tension on the deltoid muscles.

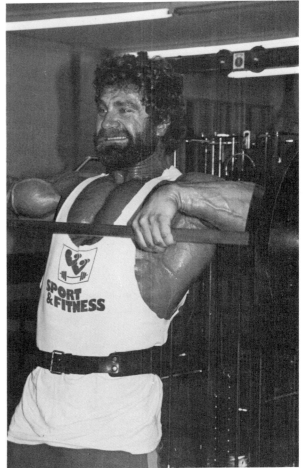

Illus. 52.   Upright row (finish).

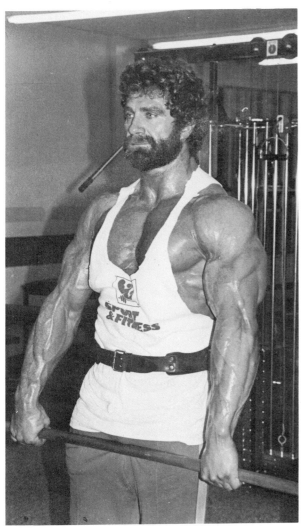

Illus. 51.   Upright row (start): performed by Jusup Wilcosz.

Two-Hand Dumb-bell Press

This may be performed either seated or standing. Start with the dumb-bells held at shoulder level, palms facing inward. Press the weights simultaneously overhead, lower and repeat.

A variation of this exercise is the "Arnold" press, which I first saw performed by Larry Scott, two years before Arnold had started weight training. This variation is commenced with the dumb-bells held at the shoulder, but knuckles facing forward (as though you had just curled the weights).

As you begin to press upwards, the movement in this particular variation involves twisting the wrists so that the knuckles twist from facing frontwards to the full twist position when they end up back-to-back at the conclusion of the press, as the dumb-bells are at arm's length above the head. Lower and repeat.

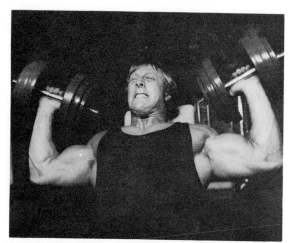

Illus. 53.   The start of the two-hand dumb-bell press, demonstrated by British great Tony Emmott.

Illus. 54.   Two-hand dumb-bell press (finish).

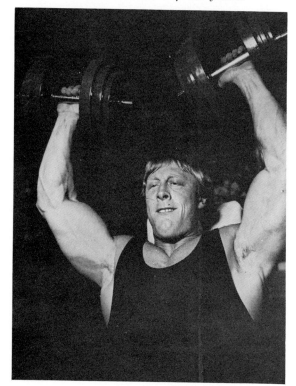

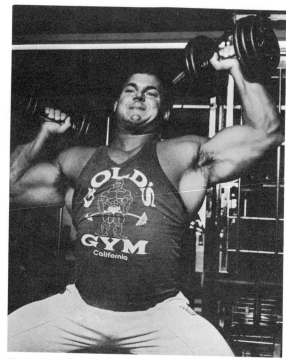

Illus. 55.   Start of the alternate dumb-bell press, demonstrated by Herculean Tim Belknap.

Illus. 56.   Finish of the alternate dumb-bell press.

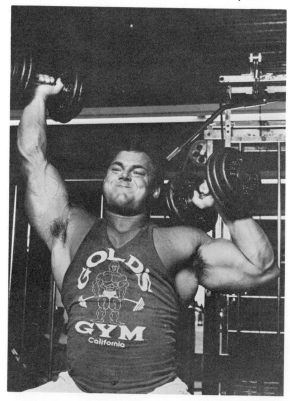

Alternate Dumb-bell Press

This exercise too can be performed in either the standing or sitting position. Simply raise first one dumb-bell, then the other in an alternating style.

This exercise differs from the two-handed version in that the body is *not* inclined to lean back during the performance, which is definitely the case in the regular dumb-bell press.

Lateral Raise

Seated or standing, the lateral raise can be performed effectively in numerous ways. You may experiment to find out which way is most effective for you.

If you are in the dark, one proven method is to start with two dumb-bells held in front of the thighs (side by side, touching). Raise the dumb-bells out to the side, keeping the arms slightly bent as you do so. As the dumb-bells rise upwards, turn the wrists downwards, as though you were pouring water out of the end of the weight (little fingers uppermost). Lower and repeat. You may work one arm at a time if you wish, as Tom Platz does or as Roy Callender does with a cable.

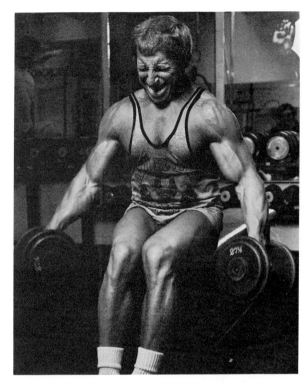

Illus. 57. Superstar Dennis Tinerino has always been known for having the ultimate in shoulder impressiveness.

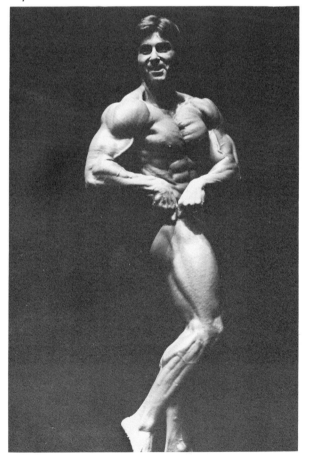

Illus. 58.   Caught in action: Ed Guiliani begins the lateral raise.

Illus. 59.   Ed concludes the motion.

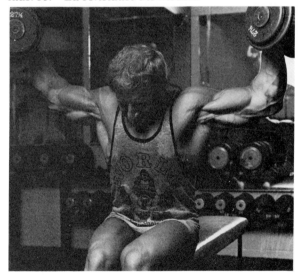

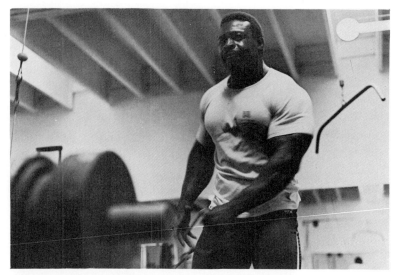

Illus. 60. Massive Roy Callender performing laterals with a cable.

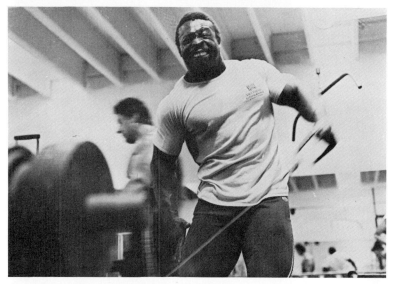

Illus. 61. The middle part of the lateral raise.

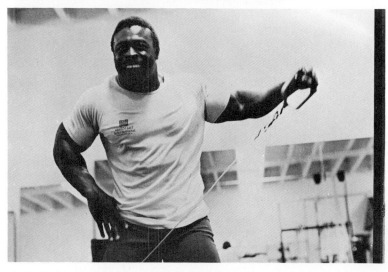

Illus. 62. Conclusion of cable lateral raise.

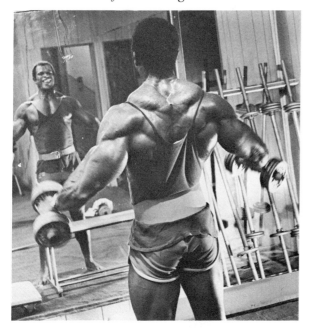

Illus. 63.   Serge Nubret performs standing laterals (start).

Illus. 64.   Finish of the standing lateral raise.

Bent-over Flying

This may be performed seated on the end of a bench, or merely in the bent-over position. Try to keep the body more or less parallel to the floor. Raise the dumb-bells upwards as high as possible and lower slowly. The arms should be bent slightly at the elbow throughout the movement. Raise and lower slowly.

Illus. 65.   Tony Emmott begins the bent-over flying exercise.

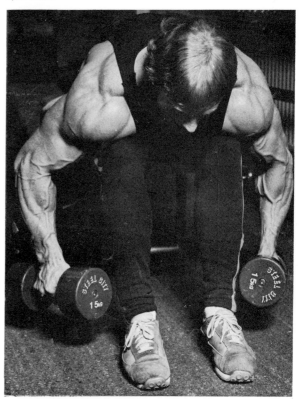

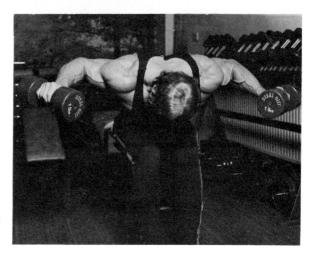

Illus. 66.   Tony Emmott shows the conclusion of the bent-over flying.

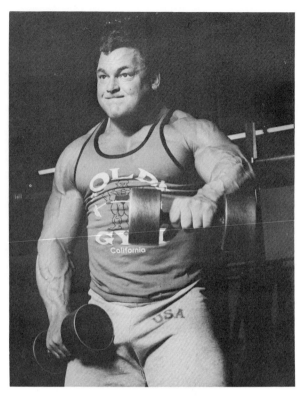

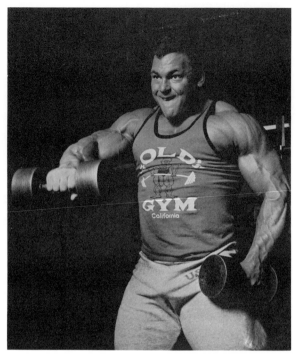

Illus. 68.   Conclusion of the alternate dumb-bell forward raise.

Illus. 67.   Tim Belknap begins the alternate dumb-bell forward raise.

Alternate Dumb-bell Forward Raise

Holding two dumb-bells, alternately raise one, then the other, straight forward until each is taken past the horizontal position. This exercise works the anterior (frontal) area of the shoulders.

Nautilus Rear Delt Machine

The posterior deltoids may also be worked using the Nautilus rear delt machine. Clench the fists strongly and push back firmly with the elbows against the pads. Return and repeat.

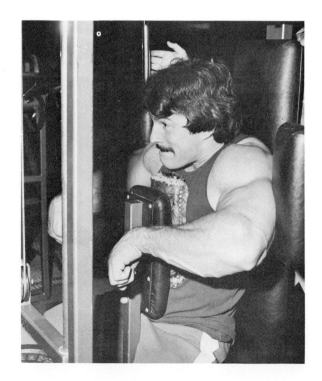

Illus. 69.   Mike Mentzer often uses the Nautilus rear delt machine for his posterior deltoids.

Neck and Trapezius 12

Very little thought is given to building the neck and trapezius. In truth, many men do not need to pay special attention to this area because most exercises involving weights do contribute, to a great or lesser extent, to the development of this region. And if you are one of those "types" that have a fairly large head (anything over 23 inches could be considered large), then in all probability in hard training your neck will already be pretty well developed as will the trapezius. If you possess a short neck, added trapezius size could possibly detract from your appearance. It will make you appear "hunchy" and give the impression that you have no neck at all!

Remember that every time you squat, row in either the upright or bent-over position, curl, deadlift or chin, you are vigorously exercising both the neck and the trapezius muscles. This may be enough stimulation to maintain proportionate development of the area.

On the other hand, if you are the tall, rangy type of person, with a long neck, possibly possessing wide shoulders, you will probably need to work your neck and traps like any other muscle part.

The traps are those sloping muscles which show themselves from the front as the area running from the neck to the shoulders. In fact they are a back muscle and actually cover a greater part of the center of the back in addition to "joining" the neck and shoulders.

Although just about every exercise you do brings the traps into action, their principal function is to draw the shoulders upwards, towards the ears.

Consequently one of the best trapezius exercises is the shrug movement. This can be performed with barbells, dumb-bells or even apparatus such as the Universal™ machine.

Have you noticed that both powerlifters and Olympic lifters have phenomenal trapezius development? The act of lifting heavy weights from the ground fully involves the trapezius muscles. They are exerted to their utmost, not solely in the upper "visible" regions, but also in the middle areas of the back. The Olympic weightlifter does a large amount of "cleans" with maximum weights and may also include a great deal of deadlifting in his training. The powerlifter, of course, has to deadlift regularly because it is one of the lifts in which he competes.

Not everybody is aware of the role of upright rowing; some believe it is purely a deltoid exercise. It is pretty well in the exclusive domain of the shoulders when performed with a 25- to 30-inch grip, but hold the barbell with hands 2 to 3 inches apart and you will find that the deltoids are involved very little. The muscle that does 90 percent of the work? The trapezius!

The ugliest pose in the book, the "most muscular" is sometimes known as the trapover or crab pose. It is the one bodybuilding pose that shows the fullest possible muscularity, particularly of the traps, because they are all but pulled out of position during the pose. Not surprisingly, the regular performance of this attitude will contribute greatly to your trapezius development.

The three best trapezius exercises follow. You need only perform one in your schedule unless, of course, you are really lacking in trap development. And as I said at the beginning of this chapter, you may not need to do any specialized trap work at all.

Barbell Shrug

Hold a barbell with a shoulder-width hand spacing while standing upright. The bar may be held in front of the body or behind, as you prefer and you may also substitute dumb-bells for the barbell.

Keeping the arms locked, raise the shoulders upward toward the ears, as high as possible. Then rotate them backward and down. Do not bend the knees and concentrate only on the up/down rotation of your shoulders. Some bodybuilders use a Universal bench press machine instead of free weights in this exercise. The "shrug" is considered to be the best all-round trapezius-building movement.

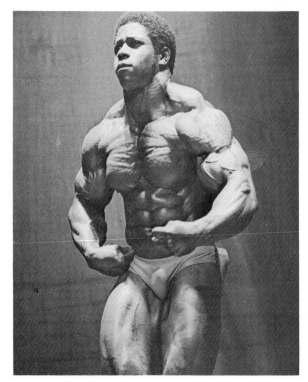

Illus. 70.   Bertil Fox flexes up.

Illus. 71.   Mike Mentzer begins the shrug.

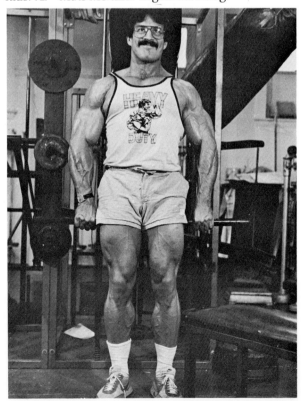

Illus. 72.   The finish of the shrug.

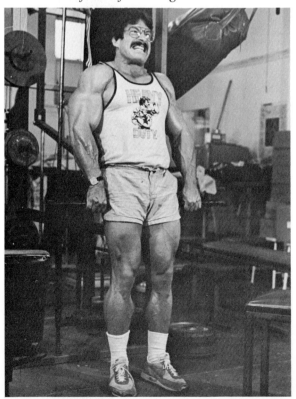

Upright Rowing

Hold a barbell with a narrow hand spacing (2 to 3 inches apart), while standing upright with arms hanging down in front of the body. The palms of the hands should be facing inward towards your upper thighs.

Raise the weight upwards, being careful to hold the elbows as high as you can throughout the movement. Lower slowly and repeat.

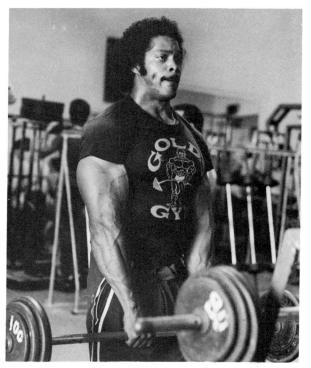

Illus. 73. Sensational Larry Jackson begins the upright row.

Illus. 74. Finish of the upright row.

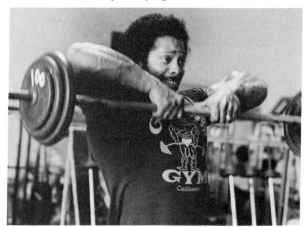

The Dead Lift

This lift or exercise starts with the barbell resting on the floor.

Take a grip slightly wider than shoulder width, one hand curled under, one hand curled over. Stand with your legs comfortably apart, with the bar almost touching the front of your lower legs. Now, bend the knees, flatten the back, hold your head as high as possible and lift the bar from the floor.

Be sure that the hips and legs take on the greatest role in the lift. Make sure that the back is flat and head is held high as you straighten up. Lower slowly, still maintaining back and head positions, and repeat. After some practice you will soon be able to use quite heavy poundages in this exercise.

Most trapezius exercises do involve the neck also. There are, however, specific neck movements you can do with the help of a training partner or a neck harness.

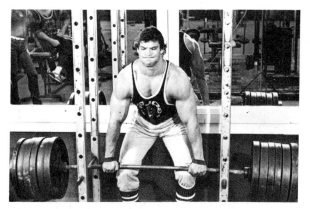

Illus. 75. David Paul begins the dead lift with what appears to be totally unliftable poundage.

Illus. 76. It's up! The finish of the dead lift.

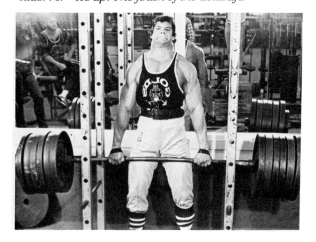

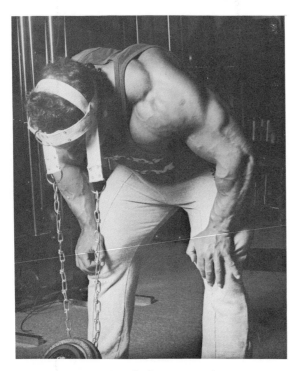

Harness Neck Raise

Stand with your feet comfortably apart, hands supporting your body, resting on slightly bent knees. Using a neck harness and weight disc, raise and lower your head through the exclusive efforts of your neck muscles. This movement can be done in reverse (for the front part of your neck). Lie on a high bench or table, with your head free over the edge. Using the same harness, with possibly lesser weight, nod your head repeatedly forward attempting to touch your chin on your upper chest.

Wrestling benefits the neck muscles greatly because the neck and virtually all muscles of the body are used extensively. The "wrestler's bridge" movement where your body becomes an arched bridge between your head and feet is very demanding on your neck muscles also, hence the huge neck development one finds on pro and amateur wrestlers alike.

Illus. 77.   Beginning the harness neck raise as shown by the incredible Tim Belknap.

Illus. 79.   The trapezius development of Serge Nubret is nothing less than sensational.

Illus. 78.   End position of the harness neck raise.

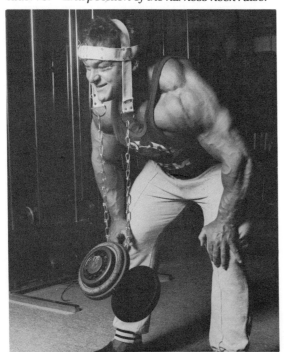

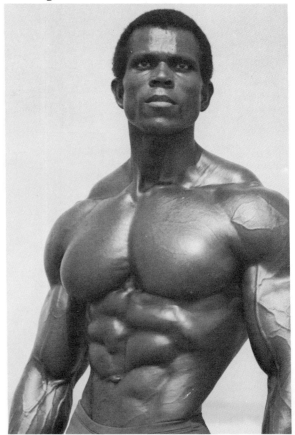

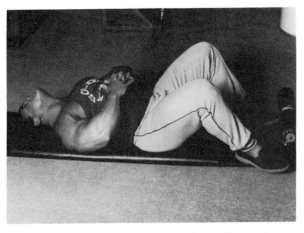 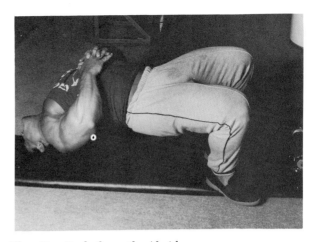

Illus. 80.   Start of the wrestlers' bridge. Belknap shows how.

Illus. 81.   End of wrestlers' bridge.

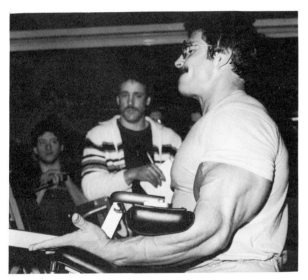 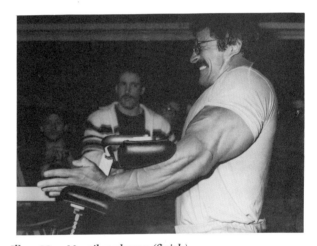

Illus. 83.   Nautilus shrugs (finish).

Illus. 82.   Mike Mentzer also uses the Nautilus machine to perform shrugs (start).

Biceps 13

Ask anybody, male or female, to show you their muscles and they'll lift up their arm and "pop" their biceps muscle. It is *the* show muscle of the body, probably the most impressive, along with the abs, of them all.

The action of the biceps is principally to draw the lower arm to the upper arm, although in the case

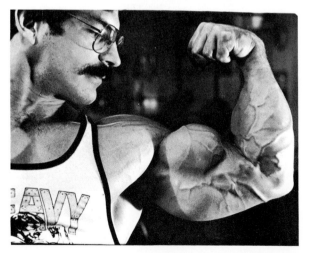

Illus. 84.   Take a look at this hard "honest" arm of heavy-duty advocate Mike Mentzer.

of chinning, the upper arm is drawn to the lower arm. The biceps also aid in rotating the lower arm as one might in looking at one's wristwatch or even drinking from a glass of water.

The most potent movements for building the biceps are those which involve curling motions. There are lots of variations. After the triceps, there are probably more exercises for the biceps than any other body part. There are numerous gadgets and gimmicks designed specifically for building biceps. The Weider Company has patented a product called an arm blaster which hangs by a belt from the neck and acts to prevent the elbows from moving during the act of curling. This is not to say that a curl performed without an arm-blaster is of no value. Many a 19- or 20-inch arm has been built without the use of an arm blaster. What the product offers can be summed up in one word—variation. It gives the trainer yet another option.

Muscles, especially the biceps, quickly grow used to particular movements, and it may be of great advantage to change your biceps exercises around to shock the area. When your biceps (or any muscle for that matter) are repeatedly shocked, there is less chance that they will settle into a state of nongrowth. I am not promising that variation will guarantee that you will never know a sticking point—if only it were that simple.

After a month or two on an exercise systematic change is often a way to chase away boredom, and is certainly a technique that gives results frequently, if not quite 100 percent of the time.

The Scott bench is another apparatus that holds the elbows in position, allowing only the lower arms to move. After many years of exercising with this bench set at a shallow slope or at a 45° angle, bodybuilders have come to realize that the best effect comes from using the bench at an 80° to 90° position.

Incidentally, it is simply not true that one can build a long biceps muscle by using the bench set at a shallow 25° to 40° angle. It does work the lower biceps, and you will break down more lower biceps fibres, but the ultimate building effect will not materialize in noticeably longer or fuller lower biceps. The shape you were born with is the shape that you have for life. You can increase overall size but there

will not be a dramatic change in shape. Having said this I will concede that a *great* deal of effort working on changing shape may ultimately lead to a very *slight* alteration in shape, but the ratio of effort to result is enormous and highly impractical.

The regular incline bench has proved a great aid to biceps development. It is Steve Reeves' favorite. In fact in the late 1940s, Steve seemed to be the only person using the exercise. It "arrived" simultaneously, via Vince's gym in North Hollywood and Ed Yarrick's gym in Oakland. Yarrick's gym which is now sadly a parking lot was where Reeves spent much of his early training. Ed Yarrick was instrumental in Reeves' early career. Together they experimented with exercises and apparatus. The incline bench was one of the "new" training aids which resulted from this experimentation.

Following closely on Reeves' success, using the incline dumb-bell curl, was Britain's Reg Park. He too enjoyed a lot of success building biceps with this exercise.

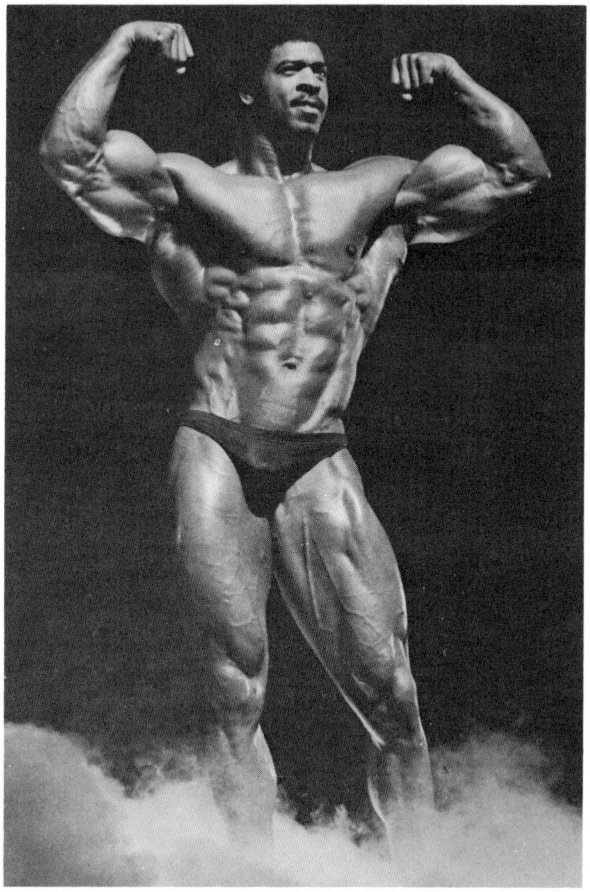

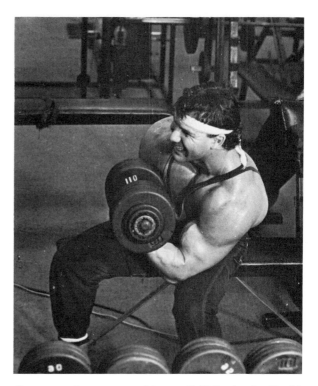

Illus. 86.   *The strongest biceps of all? Barbarian David Paul curls 110 for 10 reps!*

Illus. 85.   *Bill Grant is well known for his full, shapely biceps development.*

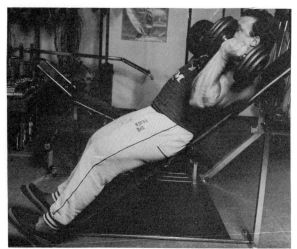

Illus. 87.   *Starting the incline dumb-bell curl.*

Illus. 88.   *Completing the incline dumb-bell curl.*

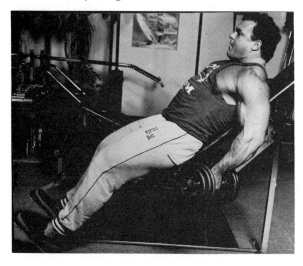

The Incline Dumb-bell Curl

Lie back on an incline bench slanted at about 45°. Hold two dumb-bells in the arms-down position. It does not matter whether you start the movement with your palms facing inward or upwards. The only difference is that the forearms are brought more into play when the palms are facing inward.

Keep your head back on the bench, and simultaneously curl up both dumb-bells. Your seat should not come up from the bench at any time during the curl. This will "aid" the biceps in getting the weight up, but in doing so will relieve them of some of the work. If they do less work, then how can they build up size or strength?

As soon as the dumb-bells reach shoulder level, lower and repeat. Some bodybuilders actually tense their biceps at the end of the curl when the dumb-bells are at shoulder level. It is just another way of maximizing intensity, and whether you choose to do it is up to you.

Barbell Curl

Generally considered the king of the biceps builders, the regular barbell curl has contributed to more 20-inch arms than any other movement.

Hold the bar slightly wider than shoulder width, and keeping your elbows close to your body, curl the weight upwards until it is under your chin.

There are two distinct styles of doing this exercise. You may perform it strictly (no leaning back during the movement, starting from a straight-arm position, utilizing absolutely no body motion or "swing") or cheating, which involves hoisting the weight up by turning the trunk of your body into a pendulum on which the barbell can rely for added momentum.

Both are workable methods, but most successful bodybuilders find they get best results from doing at least the first 6 or 8 repetitions in strict style and then finishing off the harder last 3 or 4 repetitions with a cheating motion.

Vince Gironda has his own way of performing barbell curls which he calls the body-drag curl. Basically, you hold the bar with a slightly wider grip than normal and lift the bar upwards (dragging against the body) instead of curling it outward away from the torso. When you have lifted the bar as high as possible, lower it and repeat.

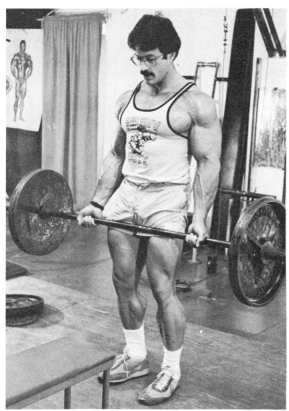

Illus. 89.   Mike Mentzer shows start of barbell curl.

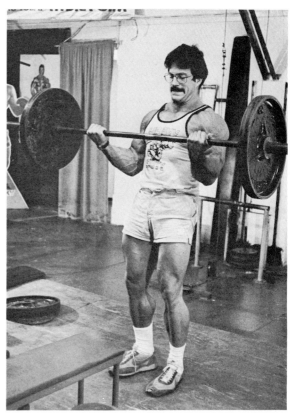

Illus. 90.   Barbell curl midway position.

Illus. 91.   Finish position of barbell curl.

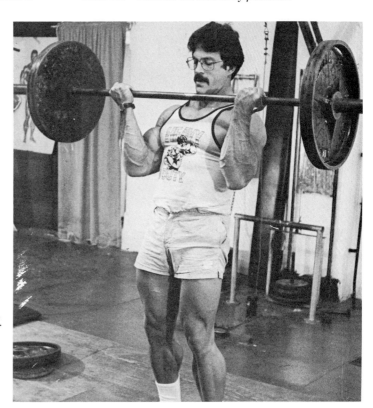

Alternate Dumb-bell Curl

This exercise is a great favorite of champion bodybuilder Rocky De Ferro. Unlike the two-handed dumb-bell curl, this movement works the biceps more directly in that the exercise prevents undue leanback or cheating. Perform the movement by standing erect and first curl one dumb-bell and then as it is lowered, curl the other arm. Lower slowly and do not swing the bells up with any added body motion.

Nautilus Curls

Place your hands carefully in position under the Nautilus pads and clench your fists. Do not begin the movement with a jerk but rather commence with a slow, deliberate, totally motivated commitment to curl both arms together. Lower and repeat. According to Arthur Jones, the creator of Nautilus, one set of maximum reps is sufficient, but that one set must contain total effort.

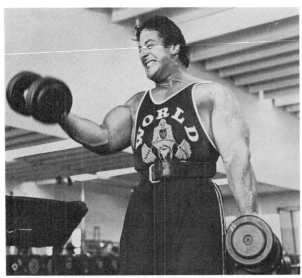

Illus. 92. Rocky De Ferro shows start of alternate dumb-bell curl.

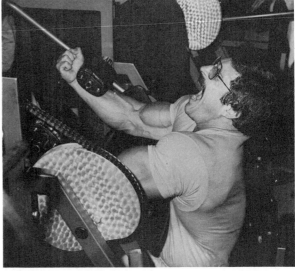

Illus. 94. Mike Mentzer at start of Nautilus curls.

Illus. 93. Finish of alternate dumb-bell curl.

Illus. 95. Finish of Nautilus curls.

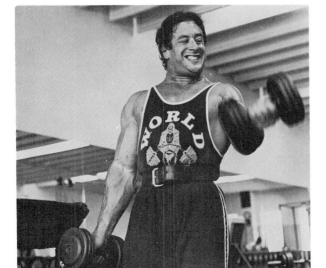

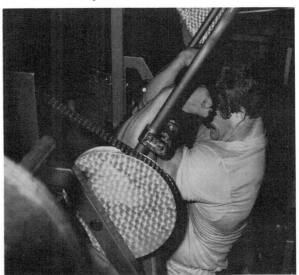

Single-Arm 45° Pulley Curls

A super finishing biceps exercise. Mr. America Tim Belknap will attest to the pumping effect of this movement. Curl the pulley apparatus smoothly and deliberately, concentrating all the time on the biceps muscle itself. If you choose to finish your biceps routine with this movement, you may perform anything from 15 to 20 reps. The pump will be unbelievable.

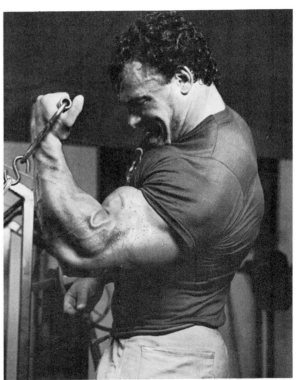

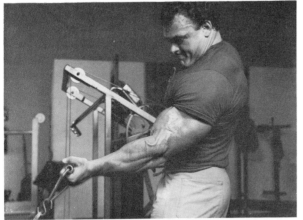

Illus. 96.   Superman Tim Belknap begins to perform single-arm pulley curls.

Illus. 97.   Tim Belknap at finish of single-arm pulley curls.

Lying Dumb-bell Curl

This is performed in the same way as the incline dumb-bell curl, except the bench is completely flat. Most people of average height or taller will have to have a comparatively high bench, so that the dumb-bells do not hit the floor at the bottom of the curl.

You may also find that this exercise puts too much stress on your arms because of the unusual position. For this reason, it is advised that you start this exercise with comparatively light weights.

Illus. 98.   Tim Belknap starting the lying dumb-bell curl.

Illus. 99.   Finish of the lying dumb-bell curl.

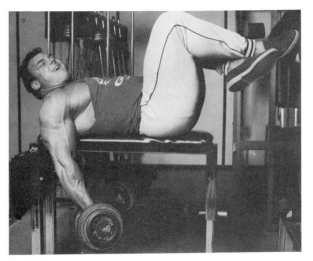

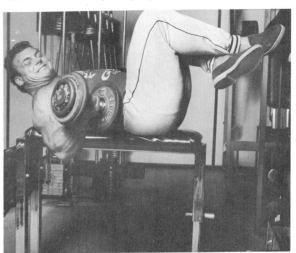

Steep Angle Scott Curls

Set the bench at 80° to 90°, making sure the bench is adequately padded so that it fits comfortably under your armpits, and affords maximum comfort for the elbows. This is important because you need to be able to concentrate fully on an exercise, and if you are in pain because of inadequate padding, you will not be able to give your entire mind to the exercise itself.

Always start each repetition with the arms straight. Under no circumstances "bounce" the weight up. This bad habit has caused many torn biceps muscles, some so severe as to have required surgical repair.

This is a favorite of Mike Mentzer's and was popularized by Larry Scott (hence the name). Previously it was known as the preacher curl or the Gironda curl since its greatest and earliest popularity came about from Vince Gironda.

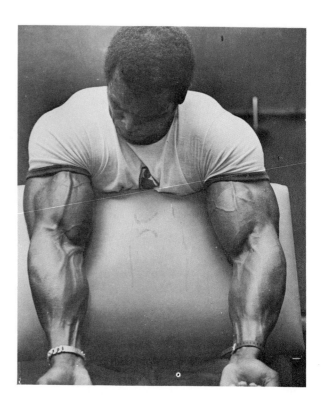

Illus. 100.   French star Serge Nubret begins the steep-angle Scott curls.

Illus. 101.   Serge Nubret at the finish of the steep-angle Scott curl.

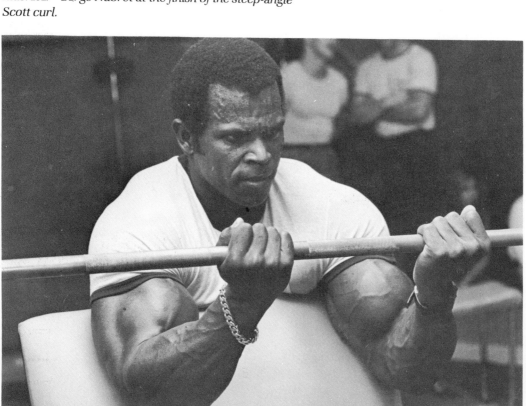

Seated Dumb-bell Curl

Sit on the end of a bench with your knees together and back straight.

Starting from the arms-hanging position, begin to curl both dumb-bells simultaneously, lower and repeat. If you have difficulty curling the weights without leaning backwards, it is a good idea to have a training partner place his foot on the bench, positioning his knee in the middle of your back. Alternatively he can sit on the bench with his back against your back. Both positions will prevent you from excessive leaning back.

If you don't have a training partner, alternately lift the dumb-bells one at a time. The mechanics of this method prevent (lean back) cheating.

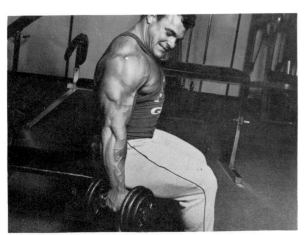

Illus. 102.   Beginning the seated dumb-bell curl.

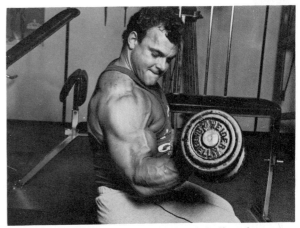

Illus. 103.   Finishing the seated dumb-bell curl.

Concentration Curl

Sit at the end of a bench resting your elbow on the inside of the thigh (above the knee). Exercise only one arm at a time, resting the nonexercising hand on your free leg.

Slowly curl the straight arm upwards and lower at the same speed. Concentrate dramatically on the biceps muscle as it contracts each time the dumb-bell is curled upwards. After training one arm, immediately do an identical number of repetitions with the other one.

Arnold Schwarzenegger has another version of this curl which he feels has contributed more to his monumental biceps size and peak than any other. He places one hand on a low stool or exercise bench, and holds a dumb-bell at arm's length hanging downwards. Arnold makes a point of keeping his shoulder low throughout this exercise. This movement which Arnold favors does in fact "hit" the biceps in an unusual fashion. It may take you a few workouts to get the hang of it, but once you do, I am sure you will benefit enormously.

Of the hundreds of other exercises for the biceps, the above are, in my opinion, the best.

There has been much discussion about the act of twisting (supinating) the hand as a dumb-bell is curled upwards. Arnold Schwarzenegger was one of the first people to popularize the theory that this action, as a movement dependent upon the biceps, would contribute to added biceps height. Arnold really believed that twisting the wrist as the dumb-bell curl was completed would help his biceps development. What he neglected to conclude was that the simple act of twisting the wrist, even when holding a heavy dumb-bell, could not possibly do anything for the biceps, unless of course, it was done against significant resistance.

Now, if the inner side of the dumb-bell was loaded with considerably more weight than the outside you would have some extra resistance during the supination. Alternatively if you held the dumb-bell unevenly, allowing as much space as possible between your little finger and the weight discs, that too would afford resistance for the twisting and could feasibly contribute towards development of the biceps.

There has been a tremendous controversy over whether or not there is such a thing as a biceps exercise that actually helps build height, sometimes known as peak. Again, let me remind you that biceps shape (what we are talking about when we consider degrees of peak) is not something that is receptive to any appreciable change. You can plump up the bundles of fibres within the biceps muscle which will increase the overall size of the area, but there is very little you can do to improve biceps height. The more positive movements include concentration curls, 90° Scott bench curls, and plenty of posing of the biceps themselves, but all in all only minor change will result.

One thing of course that does improve biceps peak is to lose every bit of fat possible from the area. You will, no doubt, have noticed that fat people or bodybuilders who have overbulked their bodies do not possess biceps peak. This is because the covering of fat "flattens" out the muscle. An analogy could be drawn with what happens to rugged terrain when it is covered with a generous layer of snow. The entire landscape smooths out. So it is with your arms. The fat fills in between your biceps and your shoulders, and in the crook of your elbows. Voilà! Unimpressive biceps peak!

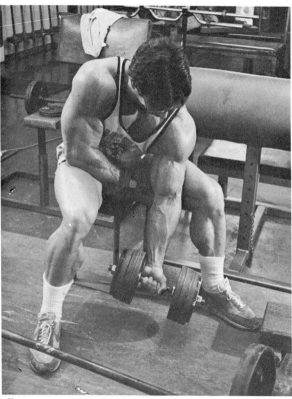

Illus. 104.   Mike Mentzer begins the concentration curl.

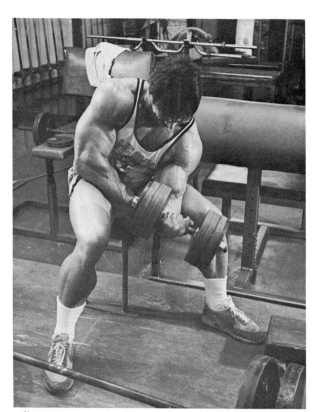

Illus. 105.   Finish of concentration curl.

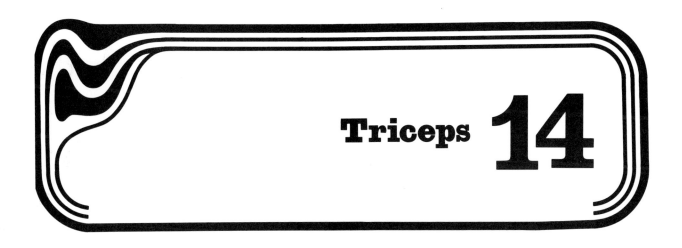

Triceps 14

There are more exercises that work the triceps muscle, that three-headed muscle situated at the back of the upper arm, than any other body part. "Triceps" in Latin means "three-headed," an inner, outer and middle head. The function of the triceps is to straighten the arm and also to bring the upper arm into the body.

As I intimated earlier there are hundreds of triceps exercises, but bodybuilders, ever searching for the movement that is *most* effective, have concluded that the best triceps exercises are:

a) Close-Grip Bench Press
b) Lying Triceps Stretch
c) Parallel Bar Dips
d) Pressdowns on Lat Machine
e) Single-Arm Dumb-bell Triceps Stretch
f) Bent-Over Triceps Extensions
g) Triceps Rear Bench Dips.

Of course there are scores of other favorites. Some bodybuilders swear by Close-Hand Floor Dips, others like using the Incline Bench Dumb-bell Triceps movement, the Triceps Barbell Kickback, Nautilus Triceps Extensions . . . the list is endless.

Curiously the E-Z curl bar was invented for exercising the *biceps* muscle. Ironically, it is used today far more often in professional gyms by those wishing to build the *triceps*. Bodybuilders have found that the middle part of the E-Z curl bar is ideally slanted to permit a relatively close grip in utmost comfort when performing standing or lying triceps

exercises. The bend of the bar prevents the hands (especially when sweaty and moist) from sliding outwards during the performance of the movement.

It is recommended that you substitute the E-Z curl bar for all triceps barbell movements. At least give it a try. If you don't find your triceps exercises more comfortable to perform, revert back to the regular straight bar.

The triceps group is extremely strong and when fully developed can endow you with enormous arm strength and substantial size. Well-built triceps can add 4 or 5 inches to your arm size.

One important aspect of triceps building, which you might not want to consider unless you personally had suffered it is elbow injury. This can occur from three incorrect training procedures:

1. Using too heavy a training load
2. Bouncing the weight in a clumsy cheating style
3. Failing to warm up.

Literally thousands of bodybuilders, in their haste and enthusiasm to build 20-inch arms, have injured their elbow joints, which ultimately adversely affected their training because of the excessive pain associated with the injury. How ironic that in their enthusiasm these bodybuilders have accidentally sabotaged the size they so desperately want. The lesson, of course, is to stress the muscle and not the elbow joint. Be content to add just five pounds to the bar each time your strength progresses. Do *not* rush things. The triceps muscles can often handle huge poundages, but the joints cannot. The most precarious triceps movements of the elbow joint are:

    a) The Single-Arm Triceps Dumb-bell Extension
    b) The Lying Triceps Stretch
    c) Triceps Pushdowns on Lat Machine.

Probably the safest triceps movements are the close-grip bench press and the parallel bar dip.

If you suffer elbow pain, it is imperative that you cease all exercises that give pain during their performance. You may find that it is simply a matter of using a lighter weight, or perhaps changing the grip or hand spacing. (Using the French grip, where the palm is facing down towards the floor in all exercises except the pushdowns on lat machine when it faces upwards, may alleviate painful elbow problems.)

At any rate, look for a substitute variation that will give your triceps a good workout without causing pain. In this way the elbows will be given a chance to mend. If you choose later to return to the exercise that you suspect may have caused the discomfort, at least observe the basic principles of good exercise style and adequate warm-up, and don't expect to use monumental poundages which could have been one of the culprits in your injury in the first place.

You will want to develop your triceps to the limit, but one has also to do justice to the rest of the body. Therefore, it is a good idea to limit the number of exercises you perform. A beginner to bodybuilding, for example, would normally only incorporate one direct triceps movement into his training schedule. Intermediates, those who have been training nine months or more, may use two triceps movements and an advanced man could use up to four different triceps movements each time he trains the area.

The usual, and proven, practice is to substitute one of the exercises now and again to break the monotony and prevent "sticking points"—which often happen when the body gets used to a certain exercise or group of exercises—the individual falls into a training rut. Then a change of exercise pattern is in order. Usually individual exercises are changed, but some champion bodybuilders break the dreaded sticking point by increasing sets. Jack Delinger, a famous past Mr. Universe would break a sticking point by doubling his reps from 10 to 20 for a few weeks and then reverting back to normal after he had jolted his muscles into growth.

Back in the 1950's I joined a bodybuilding club in England run by Stan Chisnell. Even though Reg Park was then in his prime, Stan was acknowledged as having the largest upper arms in the British Isles, 19 inches around. (Actually Park went on to surpass this measurement a few years later, becoming one of the first men in the world to possess genuine muscular 20-inch "guns.")

I learned a great deal from this Stan who combined just two triceps exercises each workout, the Standing Triceps Stretch and the Back Press with Strands. Stan did at least 8 sets of heavy bench presses each workout, and made no bones about the fact that he believed this heavy bench work contributed considerably to his triceps size, as well as his huge pectorals.

Stan would do 5 quality sets of fairly heavy Triceps Stretch movements, using about 10 reps each set, after which he would get his famous rubber cable set out and "toss" the cables over his shoulders with the rubber strands stretched across his back, elbows tucked into his waist. From this position he would press out the cables until his arms were straight out to "crucifix" position, parallel to the ground. Stan would always "start light" using no more than three or four cables. After each set he would add a cable, until after 5 to 10 sets, the entire group of cables would appear a mass of rubber. Even though there was only room on his set of strands for ten cables, he would somehow find a way to attach more. By the time he was finished the pump was superb. The cables would go back into his training bag and Stan would mosey off to the washroom, which housed the one and only mirror in the building. Sometimes when Stan felt he had obtained a really outstanding pump, he would invite a few of us skinny guys "to have a little look." We would just stand there, boggle eyed and open mouthed as he flexed his ponderous arms from several different angles, murmuring to himself, something about "feeling pretty good." Heck, we knew he felt "good." His arms were almost 10 inches bigger than ours!

Out of his storehouse of wisdom, I've never forgotten Stan's insistence on working his triceps *last* in his routine. "Psychologically it's a great feeling," he said, "to end your workout with a really good arm pump." He was so right.

Here's how to perform my recommended triceps movements. Remember not to perform them all in one workout.

Close-Grip Bench Press

A great favorite of Larry Scott, the first Mr. Olympia, who has said this exercise has given him more triceps development than any other:

Lie on a flat bench, face up, feet firmly planted on the floor. Take a fairly heavy barbell (E-Z curl bars are the most popular among the pros) from the racks (or have a partner hand it to you) using a narrow grip whereby your hands are only two or three inches apart. Keeping your elbows close to your body, lower the weight to your lower breastbone and immediately push upwards. Larry Scott and Dennis Tinerino both use in excess of 250 pounds in this movement, but naturally if you are new to this or any other exercise you should start using only light weights.

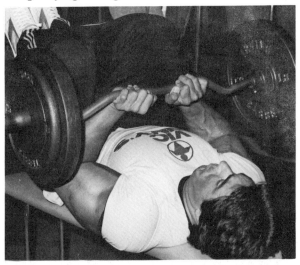

Illus. 106.   Dennis Tinerino at start of close-grip bench press.

Illus. 107.   Finish of close-grip bench press.

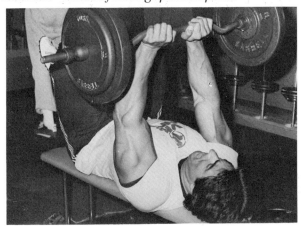

Lying Triceps Stretch

Almost every top bodybuilder owes some of his triceps size to this proven exercise. It builds bulk into the belly of the triceps.

Lie on a bench, face up. Using a straight barbell, with a grip slightly wider than the width of the bench, start with arms straight, pointing upwards. Slowly lower the weight by bending at the elbows only. Take the bar down to just behind the head, being careful not to "pin" your hair, until the bar lightly kisses the bench. Do not bounce it heavily. Return the weight to arms-straight position, trying to keep the elbows in at all times. Lower and repeat.

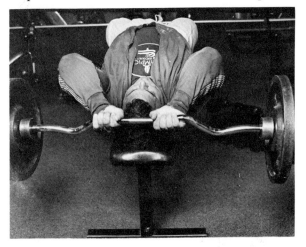

Illus. 108.   Tim Belknap starts lying triceps stretch.

Illus. 109.   Belknap finishes lying triceps stretch.

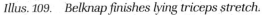
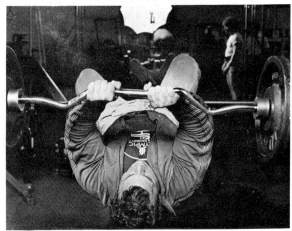

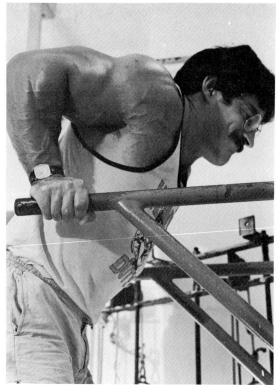

Illus. 110. *Parallel bar dips (start) performed by Mike Mentzer.*

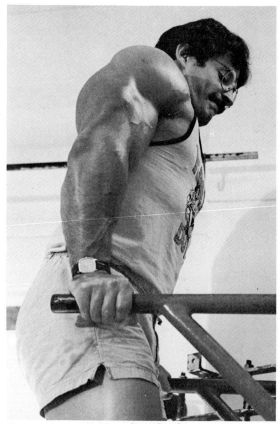

Illus. 111. *Parallel bar dips (finish).*

Parallel Bar Dips

Mike Mentzer endorses this exercise. Start with arms straight, feet tucked up under the torso, and lower (dip) while keeping elbows close to the body. Raise and return. As you get strong enough to perform 10 or 12 repetitions, then weight should be added, either by "holding" a dumb-bell between the thighs, crossing feet at the ankle, or by attaching iron discs to a special "dipping belt" designed especially for the task.

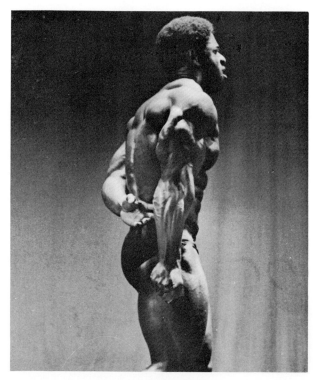

Illus. 112. *Does anyone have triceps like those of Bertil Fox?*

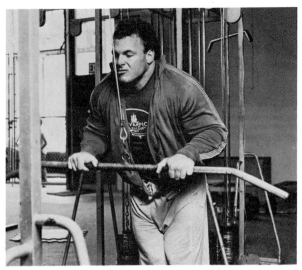

Illus. 113.   Rugged Tim Belknap starts pressdowns on lat machine.

Pressdowns on Lat Machine

Was there ever a bodybuilder who didn't spend a great deal of time and effort performing this exercise?

Start by holding a lat machine bar with hands two to eight inches apart. Now press downwards until the arms are straight. Return and repeat. Most bodybuilders keep their elbows at their sides during this movement. A few (Dennis Tinerino) deliberately hold the elbows out to the sides and "lean" more into the exercise. The choice is yours.

Illus. 114.   Finish of pressdowns on lat machine.

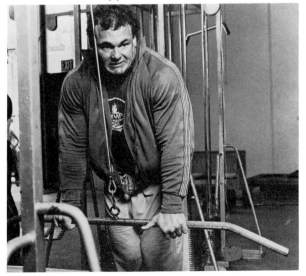

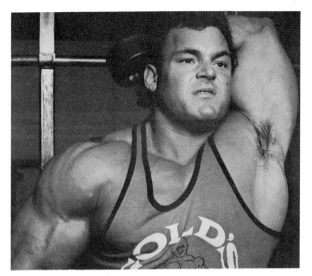

Illus. 115.   Tim Belknap begins single-arm dumb-bell triceps stretch.

Single-Arm Dumb-bell Triceps Stretch

Kal Szkalak favors this triceps exercise. It gives development especially in the lower triceps area. Although it is possible with practice to handle very heavy poundages (some top bodybuilders use over 100-pound dumb-bells), it is not always advisable to use excessive weights in this particular movement because they can put too much strain on the elbow joints and the surrounding ligaments. Beware of bouncing the weight out of the "low" part of the movement: This too can cause elbow problems.

Illus. 116.   Finish of single-arm dumb-bell triceps stretch.

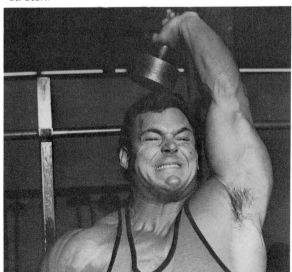

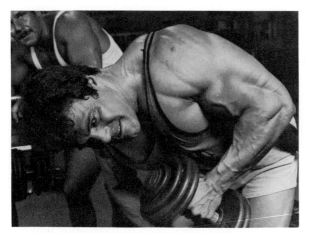

Illus. 117. *Canadian colossus Reid Schindle starts the bent-over triceps exercise.*

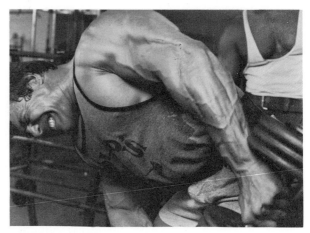

Illus. 118. *Finish of bent-over triceps extension.*

Keeping the upper arm close to the head, lower the dumb-bell behind the head, and return. Lower and raise at approximately the same speed.

Bent-Over Triceps Extension

Another Larry Scott favorite: Lean over so that the upper body is parallel to the floor. Hold a single light dumb-bell in the hand and keeping the upper arm in line with the body (parallel to the floor), raise and lower the dumb-bell. Keep the upper arm locked against the side of the waist.

Triceps Rear Bench Dips

Numerous bodybuilders, Arnold Schwarze-negger among them, end their triceps workouts with several sets of high repetition rear bench dips. Start by standing with your back to a workout bench, and support the body by resting the hands behind you on the bench, about 6 inches apart. Lift your legs off the floor and support them with a somewhat higher bench. Dip down by bending the elbows as low as possible, and return. You may place a weight disc on your thighs if the movement is too easy. Go for high reps, performing two or three sets before retiring to the shower room with an almighty pump.

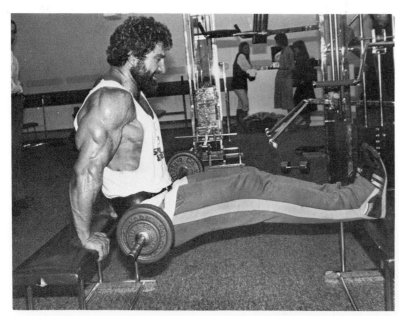

Illus. 119. *Jusup Wilcosz performs the triceps rear bench dips.*

Forearms 15

Many bodybuilders believe forearm size is supposed to develop naturally along with the rest of the physique. After all, the forearms are used in just about every exercise.

Mike Mentzer, who wields a mean forearm below titanic 21-inch upper arms, openly admits that he does not perform specific isolated exercises to develop his forearms.

All well and good for Mentzer whose genetic superiority is such that the stimulation he receives from general all-round training is sufficient to keep his forearms big and strong, but not all of us are so blessed.

Forearms come in numerous shapes and sizes, and basically the shape you are born with is with you forever. For example, if you have an "Indian club" type forearm which is typified by a long wrist with virtually no appreciable muscle development then you will not be able to change things much. Your main development will come in the upper part of the forearms.

Other people have muscles which seem to start sprouting almost from the base of the thumb. These types usually find it easy to build their forearms. They react to almost any type of strenuous physical exercise. John Grimek had such forearms.

Who has the biggest and best forearms in bodybuilding today? That distinction would probably go to Mr. America 1981, Tim Belknap. Close runners-up include Chuck Sipes, Dave Draper and Bill Pearl,

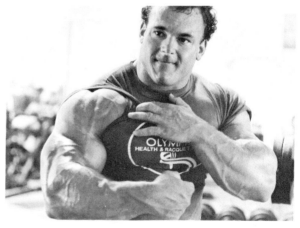

Illus. 120.   Tim Belknap—Mr. America shows his amazing lower arms.

who all train their forearms hard with isolated exercises.

It is generally considered that the forearms (along with, perhaps, the calves) are the hardest part of the body to develop. Forearm fibres are denser and tougher, but like any other muscle, will respond to regular exercise.

You must train your forearms *progressively*. That is to say, you need to practice the double progression principle of increasing your repetitions *and* weight resistance. Assume you exercise normally using a 100-pound weight for 10 repetitions. Keep pushing until after a few workouts you will be able to perform 15 repetitions or more with the same weight. Now is the time to increase the weight to the extent that you have to drop your repetitions down to 10 again. The pattern *must* be repeated. Double progression is the way to bigger muscles.

Like the calves and abs, it is generally accepted that the forearms should be worked using a system of higher reps (between 10 and 20) than for the other body parts.

Franco Columbu has some interesting thoughts on the forearms: "This is a tough muscle, not as 'pumpable' as the biceps or pecs. Forearm training has to be accomplished with virtually no rest. After a set you should pause only long enough to shake the hands, then continue exercising. It's the only way to force blood rapidly into the forearms, which in turn will bring about growth."

Some people carry hand-grip exercisers in their pocket, which enables them to work their forearms during odd times, walking to work, at the office, while waiting for a bus, etc. But there is a slight problem with the progressive aspect of such practices. You can increase the repetitions, but adding to the resistance creates another problem. One fellow I know would use his gripper with just three fingers. After a month he was down to two fingers, and so on. When he finally progresses to 20 reps with one finger, he will have to go shopping for a stronger exerciser.

As mentioned earlier, there are numerous exercises which work the forearms, but a few which work them pretty well exclusively are:

Wrist Curl

Wrist curls work the flexors (the belly) of the forearm.

Perform them in a seated position with your lower arms resting either on your knees (palms up) or on the top of a bench. Your hands must be free. Arnold Schwarzenegger keeps his elbows close while other stars allow their elbows to be comfortably apart (anything from 12 to 18 inches).

Moving only your wrist, curl the weight upwards until your forearm is fully contracted. Allow the barbell to lower under control and (like Schwarzenegger and Draper) you may allow your fingers to "unroll" to an extent, but this is optional.

Reverse Curl

Stand erect, holding a barbell at a slightly wider than shoulder width. Allow the arms to hang down straight, elbows at your side, hands overgripped (knuckles up).

Curl the barbell, keeping the wrists straight, elbows tucked in . . . lower and repeat. You will feel this exercise in the upper forearm, near the elbow.

Reverse Wrist Curl

This exercise is performed in the same manner as the regular wrist curl, the only difference being that the palms should face downwards rather than upwards. You will notice that you cannot use even half as much weight in this reverse wrist curl move-

Illus. 121.   Start of wrist curl.

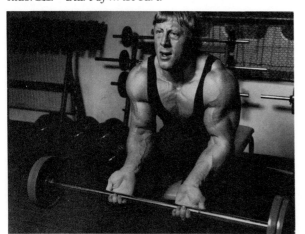

Illus. 122.   Finish of wrist curl.

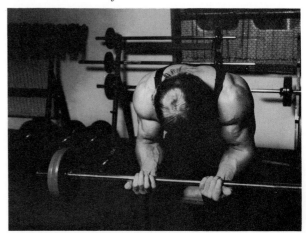

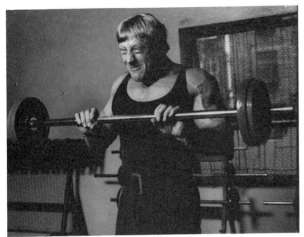

Illus. 123.   *Reverse curl.*

ment. Most people find it more comfortable to keep the arms at least 12 inches apart in this variation.

Power Gripper Machine

This machine is not very common, but it can give the forearms a very thorough workout, and allows for a comprehensive use of progressive resistance to fullest advantage.

One way to build both strength and size into the forearms is to take up nail or spike bending. It is of course advisable to start with the light-gauge metals, blunt them first to avoid accidents and prewrap the nail by rolling it in a piece of chamois leather. After practice you may be able to do more than bend 6-inch nails . . . You may be able to *break* them!

Illus. 124.   *Forearm gripper machine. Start shown by Tim Belknap.*

Illus. 125.   *Finish of forearm gripper machine exercise.*

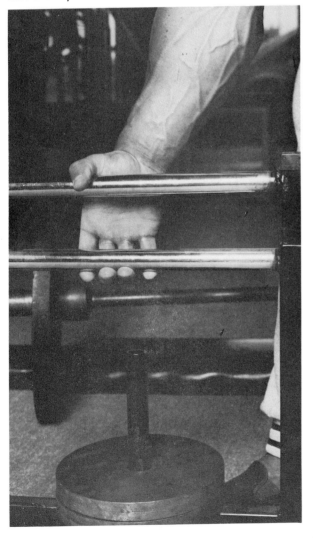

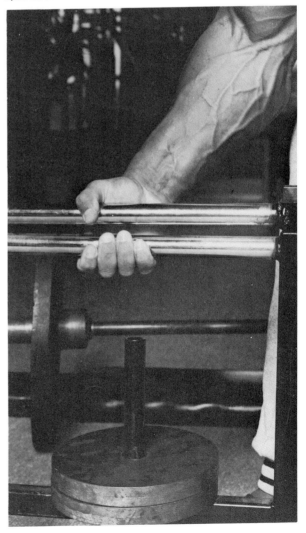

Chest 16

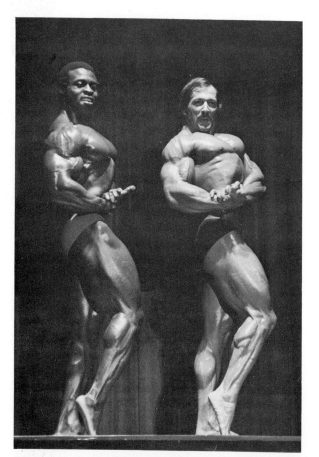

Illus. 126.   Roy Callender and Casey Viator display two of the best chests in bodybuilding.

The chest is one of the most satisfying areas to work for enthusiasts of the "iron game." This is probably because it is a pleasant area to work and is extremely responsive to regular training.

You should know right from the beginning that the line underneath the pectoral muscles is there for good. It cannot be changed. If you have rounded pecs, no amount of exercise will change that basic shape. Those with a straight line under the pecs (like Steve Reeves) are considered lucky. Certainly their shape has nothing to do with the way they train nor the exercises they use.

The chest itself can be changed and arranged to an extent, but miracles will not occur. For example, wide-grip dips on parallel bars will work the outer portions of the pectorals and help create an illusion of "flair" or width, but they will *not* make a narrow chest *really* wide.

Rib cage mobility and size can be helped by straight-arm pullovers, but a narrow chest can never be changed into a huge barrel chest. Steve Reeves could never become a Reg Park.

A skinny person with long low pecs could significantly add to his upper pecs by performing plenty of incline bench presses and incline flyes, but the upper pecs will never develop enough to make him famous for his high chest. He will always have long *low* pecs.

Those who desire huge bulbous pecs should consider the problem of *stretch marks*. If you build your pecs to a great size in a short period of time, there is a real possibility that you could also develop this unsightly condition.

Stretch marks are the result of muscle outgrowing the capacity of the skin to expand adequately to accommodate the growth. Some feel that stretch marks are only suffered by those with a vitamin and mineral deficiency, particularly of manganese. While this is as yet unproven and may be mere medical conjecture, it would nevertheless be advisable to ensure proper intake of vitamins and minerals for general well-being.

For those who already have stretch marks, there is very little you can do to rid yourself of the problem. Suntanning only helps minimally because the sun tans a stretch mark differently than a normal area of skin. There are no creams or lotions which can help. The only glimmer of hope lies in the rather drastic area of surgery, and even there total effectiveness is still in doubt.

It's easiest not to develop stretch marks in the first place, which means having patience in your bodybuilding work. Do not *blitz* your pecs too frequently, especially while overeating. The combination could give you too much chest size in too short a period, and you've got 'em for life!

Another hazard in pec building is that the muscles of the chest can be easily pulled or even torn. I strongly suggest that you warm up adequately before going all out on chest work. The pectorals (or any muscle for that matter) function better under heat. Use several pyramiding sets to build up this heat in your pecs before going to your limits. A torn pectoral muscle is not only painful, but may curtail your training for a considerable time, and can also make your chest appear asymmetrical.

Traditionally the old physical culture school of bodybuilding recommended that chest size be built from within. The battle plan was always the same: Alternate sets of heavy *breathing* squats with light straight-arm pullovers. Did it work? It worked for the fellows with naturally big rib cages who simply fulfilled their expansion potential, but failed miserably with the less-endowed ectomorphs whose narrow rib cages were not about to be expanded by anything less than the hydrogen bomb!

All forms of pullovers stretch the rib cage *slightly*. You can also help expansion by regular systematic posing: Practice vacuums, side-chest poses and chest-expanded lat spreads. In each pose consciously attempt to enlarge your cage area. Moderate success will come if you persevere. Bear in mind also that the deliberate deep breathing that accompanies and follows most formal exercise will also help maximize your rib cage size and mobility.

Bench Press

The king of weight training moves—the noble bench press—is by far the most popular exercise in the book. As you are lying on your back, feet firmly planted on the floor, a training partner can hand you the barbell, or you can take it from the rack at the head of the bench. Lower to the nipple area of the chest and push to arm's length overhead, keeping your elbows outward as far from the trunk as possible. Lower and repeat. Be sure not to let the weight bounce from the chest as this could damage the delicate nerve center beneath it. This movement may also be done with dumb-bells.

Illus. 127.   Bench press (start) performed by Serge Nubret.

Illus. 128.   Bench press (finish).

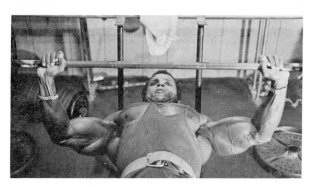

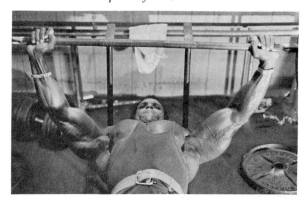

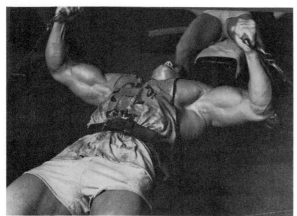

Illus. 129. *Reid Schindle starts a variation of flying—using cables.*

Flying

Lie on your back with two dumb-bells (or cables) held in the arms-straight position overhead. Lower slowly out to the side of the body (arms at right angles to the torso) as far as possible, raise and repeat. The elbows should be slightly bent throughout the movement, but should not alter position during the exercise (imagine your arm locked in a cast). Substantial weight can be used in this exercise after some practice. It may also be done on an incline bench.

Pulley Crossovers

Most gyms have pulley crossover apparatus, although the item would be considered a luxury in a home gym setup. Properly applied, the cable crossovers can enable you to work the center area of the chest in a way difficult to reach with any other

Illus. 131. *Roy Callender commences the pulley crossover.*

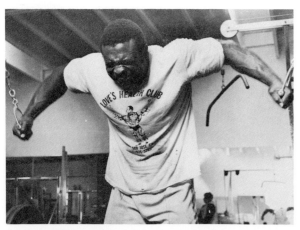

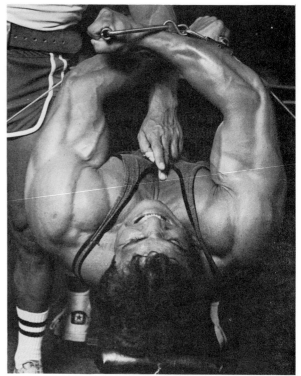

Illus. 130. *Here Reid shows the finish of the flying motion with cables.*

Illus. 132. *Finish of the pulley crossover.*

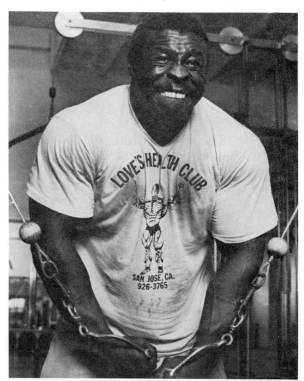

form of exercise apparatus, except perhaps the Pek-Dek®.

Hold the pulley handles in an initial "crucifix" position and leaning slightly forward, bring your hands together in front of the body. Your elbows should be fixed in a slightly bent position (that plaster cast again). Experiment with your body and hand positions to direct the maximum amount of effort into the chest region.

Incline Press

Hold two dumb-bells (or barbells) at arm's length above the head while lying on an incline bench. Usually the bench is placed at a 45° angle, but more of the pectoral is worked if the bench is set at a shallower angle, around 35° being ideal. Keeping the arms out to the sides (elbows back) and palms facing forward, lower the weights to the chest, raise and repeat. You may also do this with a barbell machine.

Wide-Grip Dips

Vince Gironda said that the largest pecs he ever saw were on an old-time iron man, Bill Trumbo. "He never did bench presses," said Vince, "only dips."

Gironda's way of performing parallel bar dips is unique and definitely workable in that it builds the pecs out at the sides (outer line) which gives an overall impression of chest width, enhancing the general "V" shape.

Your hands should be at least 31 inches apart; if you are tall, make it 33 inches apart. Throughout the dipping motion it is important to keep feet forward, chin on chest and elbows out to the side of the body. (This is a completely different movement than regular triceps dips which, although also done on parallel bars, are performed with elbows close to the body, feet tucked under the torso and head up.)

Stretch down as far as you can and raise. You will feel the effect in the pectorals after a few sets.

Illus. 133. Bronston Austin at start of wide-grip dips.

Illus. 134. Wide-grip dips (finish).

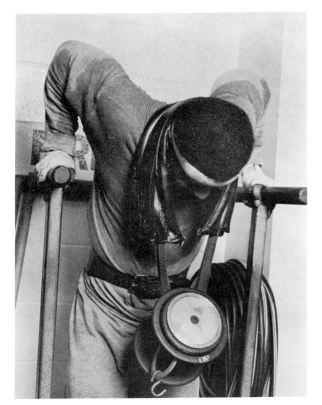

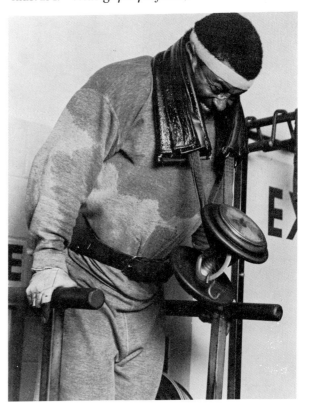

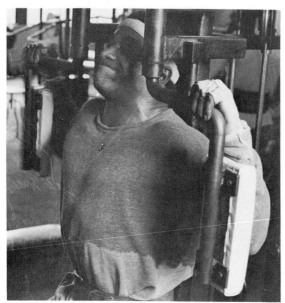

Illus. 135. *Pek-Dek crunches (start) shown by Bronston Austin.*

Pek-Dek Crunches

You need a special Pek-Dek machine for this one. Hold the apparatus securely, starting with the elbows out to the side. Concentrate hard and close the elbows together. Return and repeat. This is an isolation pec exercise and works the entire pectoral area.

Illus. 137. *Dumb-bell pullover, shown by Roy Callender (start).*

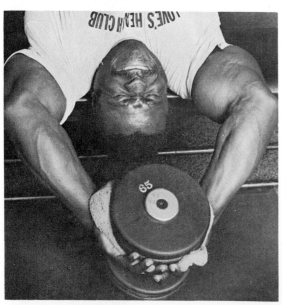

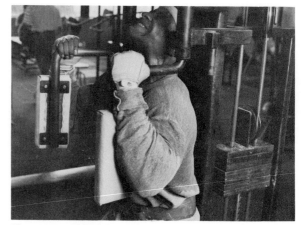

Illus. 136. *Pek-Dek crunches (finish).*

Dumb-bell Pullover

Some may argue that this is more a lat exercise than a chest movement. It does work the lat area, but credit is more often given to this movement for mobilizing the rib cage and working the upper pectorals. Start by lying across an exercise bench, supporting the upper back only. Hold a single dumb-bell in both hands above your head so that it is supported comfortably (and safely) in the vertical position. Lower slowly behind the head, keeping your arms slightly bent. Allow the rib cage to stretch fully, and return again to the arms-straight position above the head.

Illus. 138. *Finish of the dumb-bell pullover.*

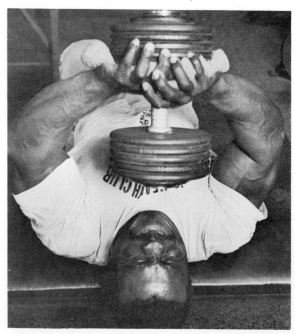

Abdominals 17

Doesn't every one, male or female, young or not so young, who cares at all about his appearance, want a lean, fat-free waistline?

Curiously, only a handful of people in a thousand actually possess such a midsection. A trim waistline is one of those elusive things that has to be well and truly earned!

I am often surprised at the number of people I meet who state an interest in "losing my beer belly" or "getting rid of this spare tire" who think that all that is needed to beat the problem is a simple exercise such as sit-ups each night. When I tell them that doing a set of twenty sit-ups each night before going to bed will do virtually nothing for the problem they seem shocked.

Waistline exercises are not the answer. Sure, abdominal movements will build and harden up the abs, *under* the flab. But they will not *remove* the flab.

So if you want clear-cut, sharp abdominal muscles, you must think either in terms of diet, or of physically burning up more calories each day. The best and fastest method is to attack the problem on both fronts. You could argue that plenty of abdominal exercises burn up calories and therefore contribute to more defined abdominals. True, but you would burn up far more calories if you devoted the time to exercises such as squats, running, cycling, swimming or rope-jumping. Abdominal exercises should be limited to being sufficient to harden up the entire set of stomach muscles . . . and then

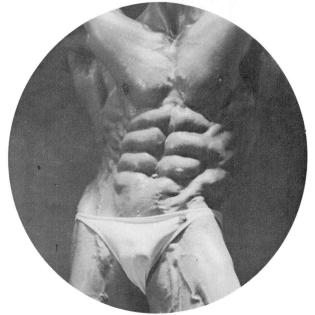

Illus. 139.

stopped. Do not try to blitz the fat away by doing scores of sets and hundreds of reps.

It is an indisputable fact, clearly understood by the world's top bodybuilders, that super abdominals are built with exercise and honed with diet.

My usual advice to people who want their abs to show clearly is to cut calories progressively, starting out the first week by reducing all sugar and sugar-loaded foods and gradually cut down on high calorie items such as beer, soft drinks, chocolate, candies, and cookies. If the fat doesn't entirely leave the area you should even reduce staple food items such as potatoes, bread and rice. A diet with all its restrictions should not be suddenly embarked upon. Rather, ration yourself with progressively *fewer* calories on a weekly basis. More advice on a bodybuilding diet can be found in Chapter 26 on definition.

Abdominals can be built up just like other muscles. Progressive resistance exercises will increase their size, but it should be understood that no amount of exercise will change their shape, or "line them up." If you have uneven abdominals, no amount of ab work will even them up and bring them into neat, straight, lined-up ridges.

Have you noticed that some really big bodybuilders have very chunky and usually noticeably bloated abdominal muscles? This is usually caused by taking anabolic steroids, often in uncontrolled quantities. Bodybuilders just do not win over contest audiences or judges with unaesthetic midsection bloat. Chunky delineated abdominals are considered a desirable feature but a waistline that is too thick, and in some cases decidedly bloated, is a disadvantage.

But Serge Nubret and Vince Gironda (who are noted for their neat, muscular midsections) keep their waists small before a contest by *not* working the abdominals during the last ten days prior to the show. "You have better control over your abs," says Nubret, "when you don't work them just before a contest. When they are not pumped you can display them better."

Your abdominal region has to be cared for throughout your bodybuilding career. One thing to watch out for is overstretching it.

Some bodybuilders allow themselves to get quite fat at times. This will not necessarily harm your ability to regain your small waistline in the future, but you should guard against overloading the stomach at any one time, because this could lead to waistline distension. Your abdominal region could be likened to a steel spring. It can be pulled out over and over again, and will return to its original position, but if it is *overpulled*, or stretched too far, it will never go back to its original shape. Consequently you should never deliberately "push out" your stomach, even for a joke. Also you should not go on marathon beer drinking (or any other liquid or food for that matter) sessions because when the stomach is overfilled, it will push outward from inside, and this too can lead to overextension.

Although a weightlifting belt is primarily designed to support the back and aid in lifting, it is also a great help to the stomach. It prevents the abdominal muscles from hanging out, especially in lifts such as squats where, during the leg and hip thrust, it is quite natural to push out the abs while completing the lift. Remember an overstretched spring does not return to normal—and neither will your stomach.

Of the hundreds of exercises for the abdominals, these are among the best. It is not necessary to perform endless repetitions, but multititle winners Bill Pearl, Frank Zane and Irvin Kozewski perform high repetitions in their ab workouts.

It is generally considered that repetitions should range between 12 and 25 and that higher reps do not bring about greater size or definition.

Incline Twisting Sit-Ups

Lying back on an incline board set at any angle you prefer (the steeper the angle the lower the part of the waist worked). Your feet should be held to the board with a strap (or bar under which the feet fit). Place your hands behind your head and curl upwards. Keep the knees bent slightly throughout the movement.

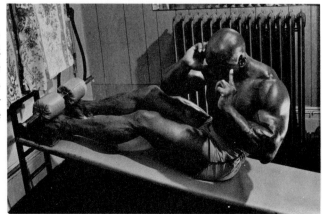

Illus. 140.   A slightly different version of the incline-twisting sit-ups performed by the "Myth" Sergio Oliva.

Roman Chair Sit-Ups

You need a Roman chair to anchor your legs in position and allow the trunk to sink below parallel, thus working the abdominal region to a greater degree. Perform this with a steady rhythm and no bouncing. This is the favorite exercise of Irvin "Zabo" Kozewski who has won more "best abdominals" awards than any other bodybuilder.

Hanging Leg Raise

Hang from an overhead horizontal bar, with your arms about 30 inches apart. Keeping your legs straight, raise them until they are just past the parallel to floor position, lower and repeat. Try not to allow the body to build up a swinging motion. This exercise works the very important lower abdominal region, right down into the groin.

For those who are unable to perform this exercise with straight legs, start off with the knees bent. Tuck your knees into the waist in each repetition

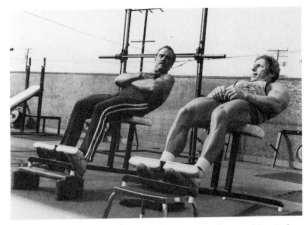

Illus. 141.   Roman chair sit-ups as performed by Zabo Koszewski and Eddie Guiliani. Zabo has performed more Roman chair sit-ups than any other person on earth!

Start the raise slowly, with positively no swinging. After a few weeks you will be able to graduate to the straight leg style.

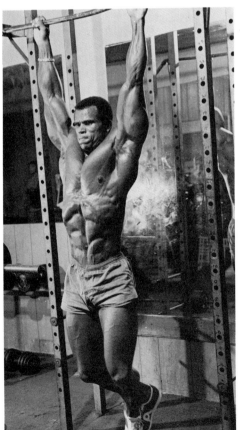

← Illus. 142.   Hanging leg raise (start) performed by Serge Nubret.

Illus. 143.   Hanging leg raise (finish). →

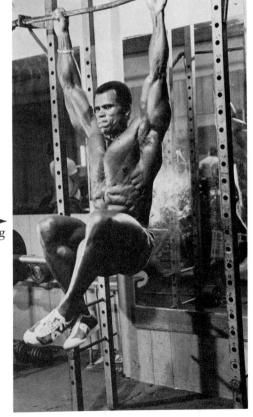

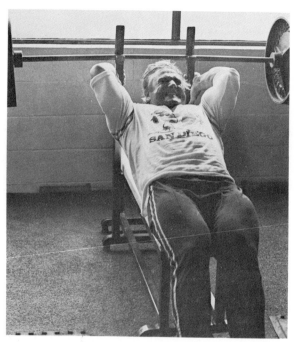

Illus. 144.   *Start of the lying leg raise as performed by Tom Platz.*

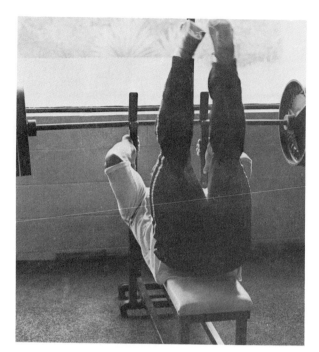

Illus. 145.   *Finish of lying leg raise.*

Lying Leg Raise

Lie flat on your back on a standard bench, holding on to the vertical uprights firmly. Keeping your back on the bench, raise your legs up from the ground until vertical. Lower and repeat. This exercise works the middle and to an extent the lower abdominals.

Crunches

Lie on your back on the floor. Your calves should rest on a bench, in such a way that your thighs are more or less vertical. Place your hands behind your head and attempt to sit up. Because of the position of the legs the peak contraction is not passed over as in the regular sit-up. There is constant tension in the middle and upper abdominals.

Illus. 146.   *Tim Belknap shows the start of the crunch exercise.*

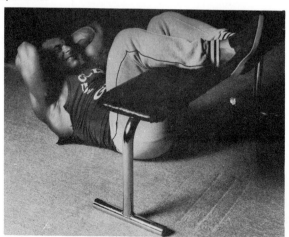

Illus. 147.   *The final position of the crunch exercise.*

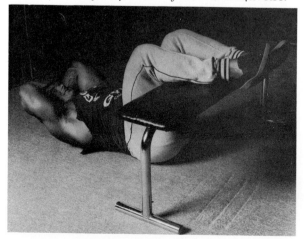

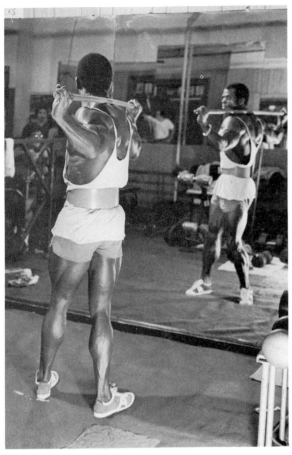

Illus. 148. Start of broomstick twist demonstrated by Serge Nubret.

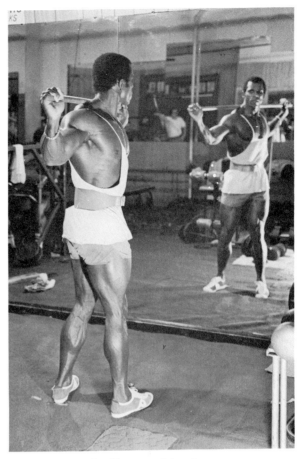

Illus. 149. Finish of broomstick twist.

Broomstick Twists

Not all bodybuilders believe in the efficacy of this exercise. It does, however, mobilize the waist area, and the obliques are worked quite strongly despite little or no resistance. Too, your ability to twist in certain poses will be greatly facilitated. Perform high repetitions as you twist from side to side, and make a conscious effort *not* to turn your hips too much to either side.

Upper Back 18

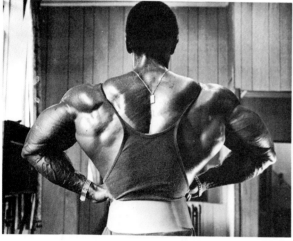

Illus. 150. The splendid back of France's Serge Nubret.

When one talks of upper back development, one usually means the "lats", known in medical and scientific parlance as the *latissimus dorsi*. The curious thing about this largest of all back muscles is that it can be seen from both the front and the back. Either way, it gives the body that important "V" shape. It is every bodybuilder's dream to bring his lats out as much as humanly possible in order to accentuate the large-shouldered, small-waisted look.

Big impressive lats are not just a product of large muscles. Spreading the scapulae (shoulder blades) by regular weight training and also by stretching contributes enormously to lat develop-

ment. In fact the scapulae can be brought out by merely pulling on a door knob with both hands, or by pulling on an upright post or wall bars. Stretch your lats several times a day like this and they will come out sooner or later. Another good way to bring them out is to perform the lat spread pose for several minutes at a time.

Of course, wide-grip chins also serve to bring out the scapulae merely by pulling outward under a great deal of strain. Contrary to popular belief, however, the lat muscles actually build more size via a moderately close grip chin because far more action is placed on the lats with this method than is obtained from very wide-grip chinning.

The other aspect of lat development is the thickening of the muscle itself which is achieved, not so much by stretching as by rowing exercises that work the belly of the muscle. Each time you are pulling (under resistance) into the waist, whether in a bent-over or sitting position, you are working the *latissimus* muscles. Vince Gironda has a special chinning method which works the belly of the lats. Using a grip on the horizontal bar about 18-inches wide, you pull your body up, not in the normal way, but until your midwaist is touching the bar! As you may imagine this is extremely difficult to do (most people cannot even do one rep), but once mastered, is a dynamic lat exercise.

Some people have "high" lats while others have "low" lats. Franco Columbu is an example of someone with low lat development and Johnny Fuller could be characterized as having high lats. Generally speaking, the shape of your lats is determined genetically. You inherit the height of your lats. Fellows with low lats should do plenty of wide-grip chins and those with high lats should concentrate on rowing exercises, pulling the weight into the tummy. A certain amount of "averaging out" will result from this training, but if your problem is extreme you will probably not rectify it completely. Recommended lat exercises are:

Wide-Grip Chin

Grasp an overhead bar using an overgrip (palms down) at least a foot wider than your shoulders on either side. (If your shoulders are 2 feet across, take a grip about 4 feet wide.)

Pull upwards, keeping your elbows back throughout the movement. You may pull up so that the bar is in front or behind your neck. This is entirely up to you. Some bodybuilders like to change around for variety, but it would not be correct to say that one form is superior to the other.

Lower until your arms are straight and repeat. Once you can perform 12 to 15 reps, it is a good idea to attach added weight with the help of a weight belt after which you can build up your reps again.

Lat-Machine Pulldowns

This exercise has to be performed on a lat-machine. Take a wide overgrip on the bar and pull down as far as you can. This exercise is not as effective as the wide-grip chinning exercise, but does have the advantage that you can use less resistance and consequently can pull the bar lower and work your lats over a greater range of movement.

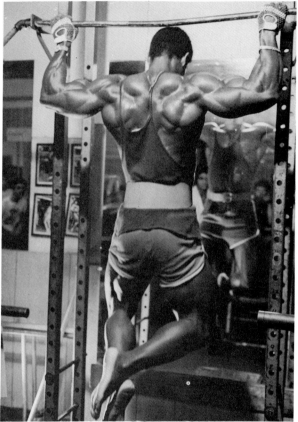

Illus. 151.   Serge Nubret completes the chin behind neck.

Illus. 152.   Start of lat-machine pulldowns demonstrated by Serge Nubret.

Illus. 153.   Finish of lat-machine pulldowns.

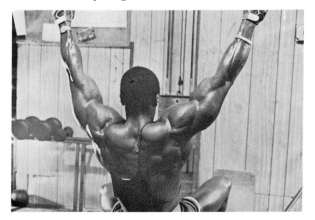

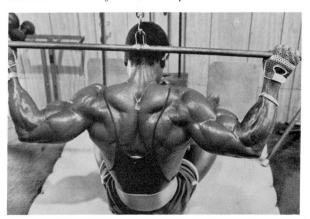

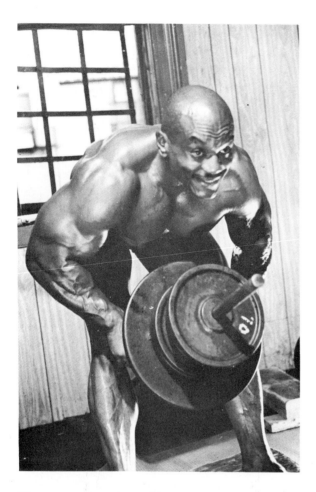

Bent-Over Rowing

This is one of the most popular exercises for putting some meat on your lats. Grab a barbell with hands about 24-inches apart. Bend your knees slightly and keep your head as high as possible while bending your torso parallel to the floor. Keep your lower back flat, your seat stuck outward, and pull up vigorously on the bar. Pull it into the tummy, not the chest. Lower until arms are completely stretched . . . and more. Do not rest the weight on the floor until the set is completed. Pull up and repeat. Some bodybuilders prefer to use a single dumb-bell, working one arm at a time. The effect is slightly different, and may in fact safeguard you from back injury, a real possibility with regular barbell rowing, especially if you are predisposed to back trouble or are using weights that are just too heavy. This exercise may also be done using one end of a bar as shown by Sergio Oliva. (This exercise is sometimes called T–bar rowing.)

Low Pulley Rowing

Perform this movement with a long cable machine. Secure your feet against the apparatus and pull the cable handles horizontally into your midsection. Hold for a second and slowly allow your arms to straighten and ultimately stretch your lats. Pull in again and repeat. You may also perform this exercise on a high pulley as shown by Reid Schindle.

Illus. 154. The indomitable Sergio Oliva performs the T-bar bent-over rowing variation.

Illus. 155. Super Gold's owner Pete Grymkowski at the finish of low-pulley rowing.

Illus. 156. Reid Schindle performing lats on the high pulley.

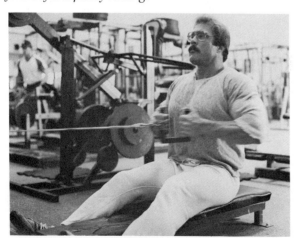

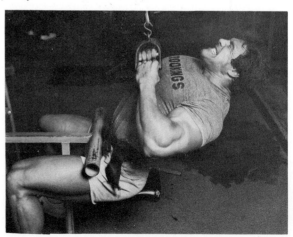

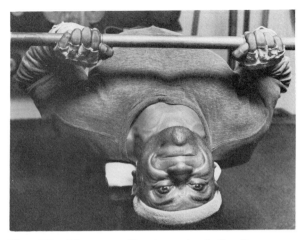

Illus. 157.   The start of bent-arm barbell pullover.

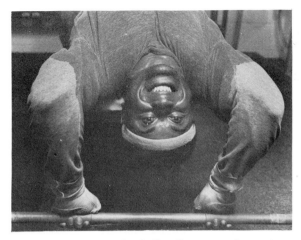

Illus. 158.   Bent-arm barbell pullovers performed by Bronston Austin (finish).

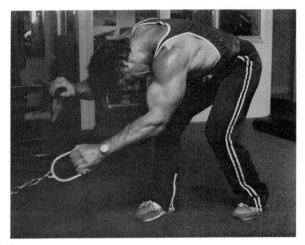

Illus. 159.   Low-pulley single-arm rowing performed by Rocky De Ferro (start).

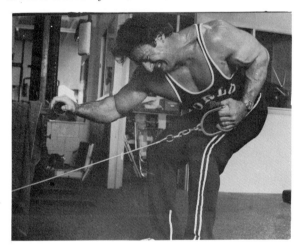

Illus. 160.   Low-pulley single-arm rowing (finish).

Low Pulley Single-Arm Rowing

Grab hold of the handle of a low-weight pulley and set yourself in a comfortable bent-over position. Starting with the arm straight, pull the handle strongly into the waist. Make the lats feel the effort strongly. Return to arm-straight position and repeat.

Bent-Arm Barbell Pullover

Lie flat on an exercise bench with your head hanging over the end. Hold a barbell with a grip of between 12 and 14 inches. Start with the bar held at the chest and lower it slowly behind the head. Concentrate on feeling the effort in the lat area. Pull back to the original position and repeat.

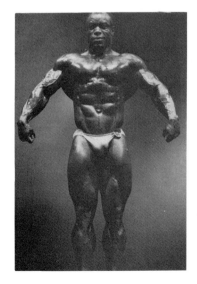

Illus. 161.   Note the high lat development of Britain's Johnny Fuller.

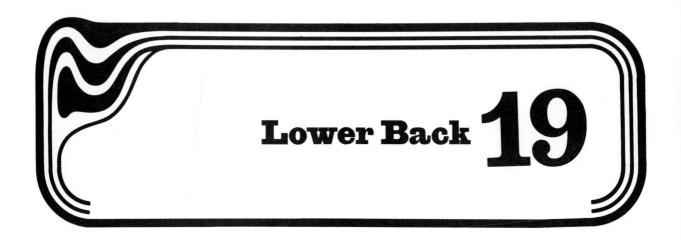

Lower Back 19

Generally speaking, the lower back is the most neglected area of the body. This is somewhat paradoxical since it is also the area referred to by physical culturists as the "seat of health."

The bodybuilder would be wise to train his lower back regularly, not only to keep the area strong and healthy, but also to build up the important lumbar muscles to gain maximum points in open bodybuilding competition.

Ten short years ago, bodybuilding judges hardly gave the lower back a second glance. Certainly no one ever lost a contest because he had a weak-looking lumbar. Today, things are different. Lower back development can make or break you. Whereas it still does not attract the attention of, say, the arms or chest, bodybuilding judges nevertheless evaluate the entire physique—and the lower back region is an important part of your body.

One of the important points about weight training for beginners is that they learn to lift a barbell from the floor correctly. This lesson, once learned, must never be forgotten, because one day a careless move can twist your back and cause a pulled muscle or, even worse, a cartilage or disc problem.

Whenever you lift a weight of any kind from the floor, bend the knees, flatten the back, stick your bottom out forcefully, and lift upwards. Make sure the weight is as close to the body as humanly possible. Many a lower back has been "strained" by trying to lift an object that is not sufficiently close to your center of gravity.

Most exercises that one does with weights involve the lower back to some extent. Perhaps that is why so few bodybuilders bother to perform specific lower back exercises. They feel that the area obtains enough stimulation from the spill-over effect of generally working out. I personally advise that one of the following movements be included in your routine. In this way your lower back will keep strong and healthy, and the muscles will always appear thick and superbly developed.

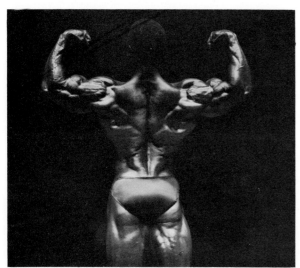

Illus. 162.   Few men have a lower back as impressive as Roy Callender's.

"Good Morning" Exercise

Place a light barbell across the back of your shoulders, and with your legs comfortably apart, lean forward at the waist. Keep the knees locked, back flat and head up. It is important that you hold tightly onto the barbell. Dip as low as possible without undue discomfort, straighten up and repeat.

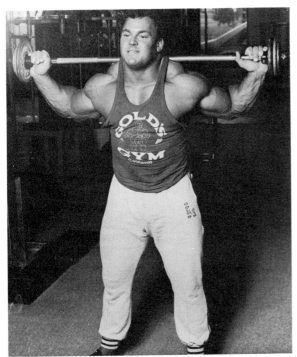

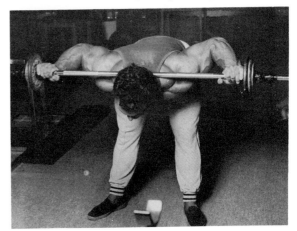

Illus. 163.   Beginning the good-morning exercise by Tim Belknap, Mr. America 1981.

Illus. 164.   Completing the good-morning movement.

The Dead Lift

Stand over the barbell with the bar touching against the front of the lower legs. Grab the bar with an alternate grip (one hand undergrip, one hand overgrip), hands about two feet apart. Bend over the bar, back flat, bottom out, knees bent, head up. Now, without bending your arms, lift the weight from the floor, until your body is completely upright. Lower and repeat, bearing in mind as you do that you must never cease to adopt this important flat-back position.

Illus. 165.   Tim Belknap starts the dead lift.

Illus. 166.   Finish of the dead lift.

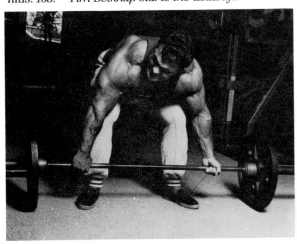

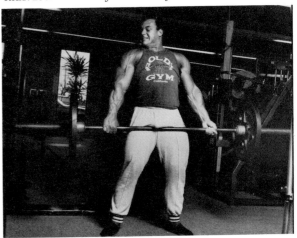

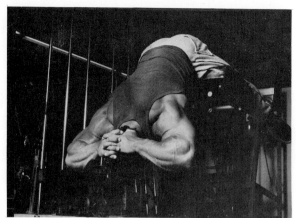
Illus. 167.   *Start of prone hyperextension.*

Prone Hyperextension

This is performed on an exercise unit especially designed for the job. Until recently, it was performed from a high bench or table. Place the legs and hips, front downwards on a suitable table top. A training partner should hold your legs down to prevent your falling off the end. The upper body should be free to rise up and down. Place your hands behind your head and lower your trunk towards the floor. Rise until your body is in a straight line. Lower and repeat. In time, as your lumbar region strengthens, you may hold a barbell behind your head as in the good morning exercise. This movement is a great favorite of Mike Mentzer's and Reg Park's.

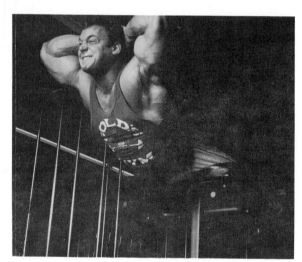

Illus. 168.   *Finish of prone hyperextension.*

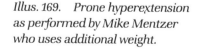
Illus. 169.   *Prone hyperextension as performed by Mike Mentzer who uses additional weight.*

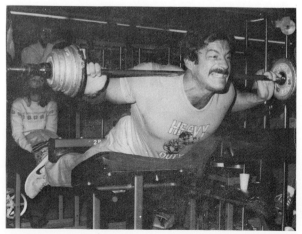

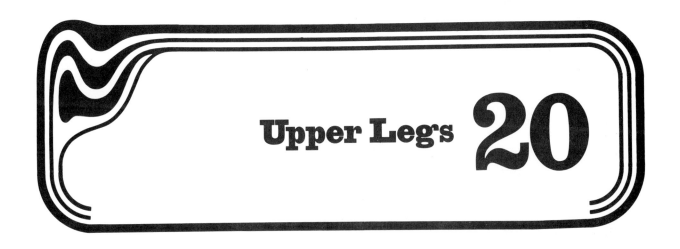

Upper Legs 20

For years bodybuilders only squatted to develop their thighs. Very few performed any other type of upper leg exercise. Basic back squats did a pretty good job until the late 1940's when men like Vince Gironda and Steve Reeves started paying more attention to the shape of the upper legs. Since the thighs are made up of different muscles, the shape can be moulded more or less as one wishes.

Vince Gironda is strongly against squats: "Heavy back squats are not part of my world. Neither do my pupils perform them. In fact, in my gym there are no squat stands because I do not want to encourage students to practice heavy squats which spread the buttocks and widen the hips."

Steve Reeves felt the same way: "I liked to perform the front squat or hack lift for thighs. The back squat concentrates the effort too much on the hips, buttocks and upper thighs."

Other opinions differ: John Grimek, the only undefeated top bodybuilder says, "I do not believe heavy back squats overbuild the buttocks and spread the hips. Most men just do not work squats hard enough to get proper benefit. And of course their hips will spread if they overeat, because this central area is one of the first to carry fat if one consistently takes in too many calories."

There is no doubt that regular heavy back squats will develop the glutes (gluteus maximus) but after all this area is a muscle, and should at least be developed to some extent. The problem lies, I feel,

with the overuse of the squat. Beginners should squat regularly, intermediates and advanced men should regulate their squatting in accordance with their development. Some may need 4 or 5 sets of squats every workout, while others may only have to squat for a couple of sets each month. Such is the variability of individual genetics.

Squats build weight and roundness into the thighs and buttock area. They are undoubtedly the best exercise for building size into the thighs. It has also been known for years that a regular program consisting of sets of progressive squats will greatly benefit overall gains. Many a trainer has ceased to gain a significant amount of muscle until he has embarked on a program of squatting. When you work the largest muscles in the body you are putting great stress on your entire constitution. Accordingly your metabolism is greatly stimulated and overall growth is promoted.

You may find that squatting is extremely uncomfortable. Certainly it is the least favorite exercise. Most bodybuilders sigh with relief after finishing their squats, which is ironic in that squats do more good than any other movement.

Here is how you can make your squats more comfortable:

1. Perform them while resting your heels on a 2½-inch-high block of wood. (Some people use books.) This will help hold your back upright and prevent you from coming up out of the squat, bottom

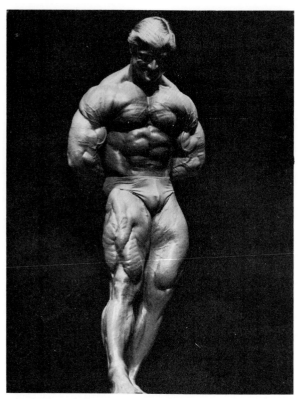

Illus. 170.   Tom Platz's legs are the phenomenon of the century.

concentrate on the task at hand rather than worry that you might get stuck in the squat position.

While squats are the number one thigh exercise, bodybuilding experts have come to realize that the thigh needs other "supplementary" movements to bring it up to full potential. Thigh curls are a must. They work the biceps at the rear of the upper leg. Other important exercises are hack slides for the lower thigh, thigh extensions and leg presses for the middle thigh and lunges for the upper frontal area.

A program for the upper legs usually consists of basic squats, thigh curls and perhaps one other exercise from the supplemental exercises.

Today, thigh development forms an important part of bodybuilding competition. Not only are the judges looking for overall size both in the upper, middle and lower regions of the thigh, but also for well-rounded leg biceps. In addition, the various sectors, *vastus internus*, *vastus externus* must be fully developed and balanced. The upper thigh must be pronounced, showing all the intricacies of development and separation. Even the abductor muscles must show as should the *sartorius* on the inner thigh. Cross-striations as seen on the thigh of Tom Platz and a handful of others when they are in top condition are also a plus in any competition.

Who has the best upper legs in the business? Certainly in days gone by Reeves was a top contender. But judging by today's standards Gironda was way ahead of his time. He had upper leg muscularity that went from his knees to his groin. Today men like Steve Davis, Chris Dickerson, Roy Callender, Tom Platz, Frank Zane, Samir Bannout and Tony Pearson have complete thighs in that they possess full development and muscular separation right from groin to knee.

A famous bodybuilder once asked me, "Bob, how do guys like Steve Davis and Tony Pearson get that thigh separation right at the top of the leg where they seem to come out from under the pose trunks?"

The answer is plenty of leg exercises, such as lunges, and leg presses, coupled with a low-calorie diet (the thinner the skin the more a muscle will "show"). But most important of all is to "pose out" the area. That is to say, you must constantly practice controlling and posing the upper area of your thighs. Place one foot 6 inches forward and press your heel into the ground, concentrating on bringing out the upper thigh. It is this, more than any other formal exercise, which will give that special look to the upper thigh area. Give it ten minutes every day and look for real results after a couple of months.

first, with your head between your knees, a most unwise habit.

2. Lower only until the tops of your thighs are parallel to the floor. Do not squat deeply and on *no* account *bounce* out of a low squat position.

3. Place the bar securely behind your neck and hold onto it tightly, hands about 27 to 30 inches apart. Really skinny guys may find that they need to pad the bar (roll a towel around the middle, or use some foam rubber) to prevent it from cutting into the upper back. This habit should be stopped, however, as you develop some muscle. You will soon learn to find a suitable resting position for the bar as you get "into" squatting.

4. If you find that you are gasping for air even before your thighs are giving out, you must develop more cardiovascular efficiency (wind). Run two or three times a week; skip rope; cycle or swim. Nothing is more uncomfortable than gasping for air with a heavy weight across your back. If you develop good wind, squatting will be far less obnoxious.

5. Always use a good set of squat racks with "catchers." If your racks do not have this safety feature, you need a training partner (preferably two) to spot you during the exercise. This will allow you to

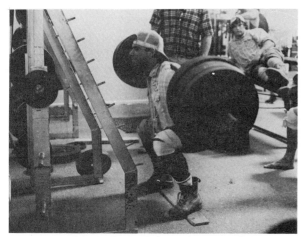

Illus. 171 and 172. *The squat (Barbarian style). 171 (above) the start; 172 (below) the finish.*

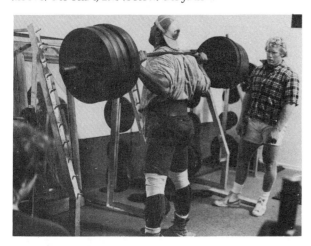

Squat

It is sometimes known as the basic squat, back squat, regular squat or formal squat; it is surely the king of all leg exercises.

Take a loaded barbell from the squat racks. After securing it behind the neck, holding the bar in place with the hands, step one step backwards from the racks and, using a block of wood 2½ inches high under the heels, squat down until the upper line of the thighs is parallel to the floor. Return to standing straight position and repeat. During the movement it is necessary to keep the back flat, seat stuck outward, and head up. All squats should be performed either in front of a mirror or a plain wall. This allows for minimal distraction and utmost concentration on what you are doing. It is important to breathe deeply during your squats. Fill the lungs with air before descending and wear a belt during the exercise.

Hack Slides

This exercise is done on a special hack slide machine. Place your feet comfortably apart and slide up and down by bending and straightening your legs. Do not handle too much weight. It is better to perform the exercise with a steady rhythm rather than use a heavy weight that may cause you to fall out of position and work the thighs incorrectly.

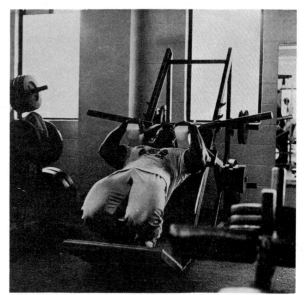

Illus. 173. *Start of hack slide shown by Canada's Roy Callender.*

Illus. 174. *Finish of hack slide.*

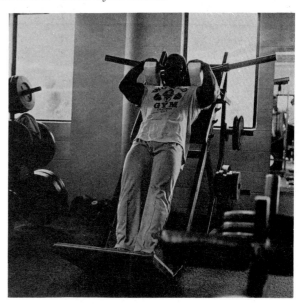

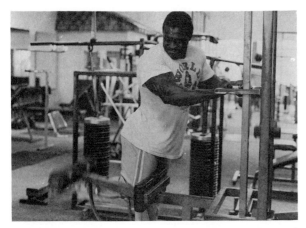

Illus. 175. *Roy Callender prefers the standing leg curl.*

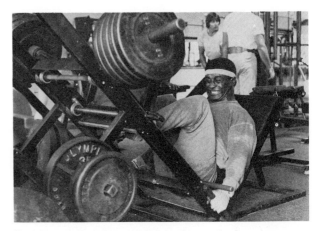

Illus. 176. *Bronston Austin performs the leg press.*

Thigh Curls

Lie on your front, with your feet about 12 inches apart. Curl up on a thigh curl machine and lower under control. Do not allow the feet to drop, but rather let the thigh biceps feel the effort as the weight is lowered. Some thigh curl machines allow for upright single leg curls.

Leg Press

This exercise is performed on a special "leg press" apparatus. Lie on your back and after placing your feet in position, press the weight upwards. Lower slowly and repeat. The leg press was designed to take the place of the squat which many body-builders find uncomfortable. Let's face it, heavy squatting can be nauseating. Unfortunately, the leg press, good as it is, does not give the phenomenal results that you get from squats. Some leg press machines are set at an angle while others are arranged so that you press directly upwards.

Lunges

Stand with feet together with a light barbell across the back of your shoulders held in position by your hands.

Step one pace forward with the left leg and bend it until the left thigh is parallel to the floor, the knee of the right leg almost touching the ground. Keep your upper body as erect as possible and return to the feet-together upright position. Next place the right foot forward and follow the same procedure.

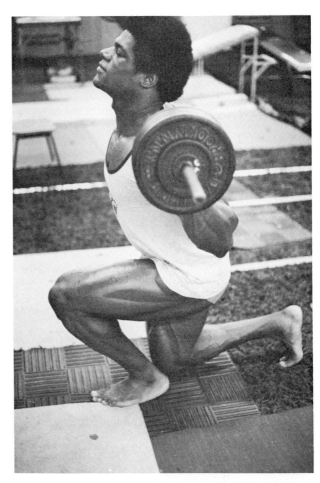

Illus. 177. *Muscle king Tony Pearson shows the lunge.*

This exercise works the entire thigh area and is particularly useful in stimulating upper thigh muscle separation.

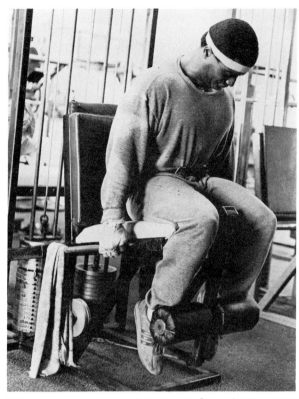

Illus. 178. *Thigh extensions (start) shown by Bronston Austin.*

Illus. 180. *The amazing Bronston Austin will perform thigh extensions using one leg at a time (start).*

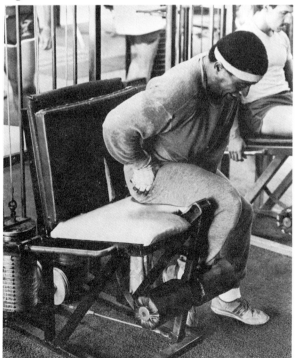

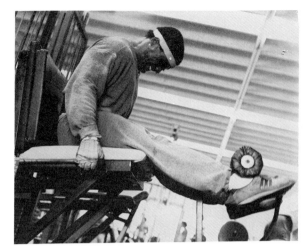

Illus. 179. *The finish of the thigh extension.*

Thigh Extensions

A special piece of equipment is needed for this movement. Slowly raise and lower the legs, concentrating on the movement at hand. Do not kick the weight up because this allows your muscles to take advantage of the momentum. If they are not made to work hard, they will not build up to the utmost degree. You may exercise both legs together or one at a time.

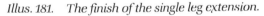

Illus. 181. *The finish of the single leg extension.*

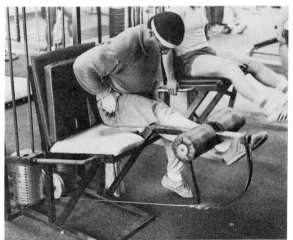

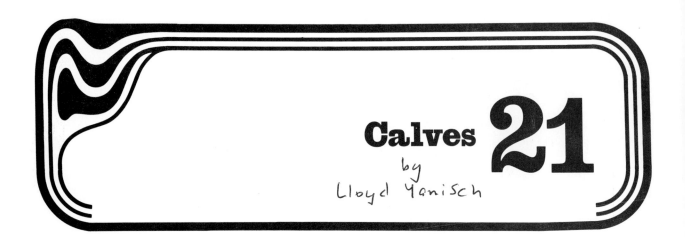

Calves 21

by
Lloyd Yanisch

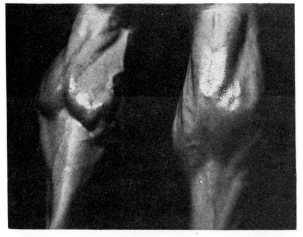

Illus. 182.   The outstanding calf development of Casey Viator.

If you've ever seen Chris Dickerson's calf close up, you will appreciate the sheer beauty of a fully developed and perfectly shaped lower leg. And what happiness to have heredity on your side when it comes to calf development. I'll never forget Johnny Fuller's answers to Chris Lund's questions on calf development. Chris asked Johnny what his calf measured. Fuller replied that it was 19 inches. "Gee," said Lund, "that's humungous! What did they measure when you first started training as a kid?"

Johnny Fuller looked Lund straight in the eye: "18 inches," he replied.

Virtually all top bodybuilders train their calves, but many have to really fight and sweat for every quarter inch, while others get by on just training their calves prior to contest time. If you have natural calves then you probably also have natural legs, and that means you can maintain those legs with minimal training, which gives you a whole lot of extra energy and time to devote to your torso and arms.

Three men who come to mind who did not have naturally big calves are Reg Park, Arnold Schwarzenegger and Lou Ferrigno. Park concluded that he would have to blitz his calves to bring them up to par with his large thighs so he worked with extremely heavy weights (over 800 pounds) on the standing calf machine, regularly, sometimes twice daily. Within a fourteen-month period, he had brought them from an unimpressive 16 inches to just under 19.

When Arnold Schwarzenegger came along in the mid-sixties as a teenager with tremendous upper body potential and unusual drive, his calves were noticeably down. When this was pointed out to him he decided to do something about it. After talking to Reg Park, Arnold chose to follow Park's method of beating the problem, which was to pound his calves two times each day with extremely heavy weights. To give Arnold his due, he did work harder on his lower legs than any man had before him. The results reflected his intense efforts. At the age of 20, Arnold's lower legs were around 16 inches. Two years later he had got them up to 19 inches, but he still persevered and at his best they measured a full 20 inches.

Lou ("the Hulk") Ferrigno was another who built an enormous body, but neglected to build his calves sufficiently. In the manner of Park and Schwarzenegger before him, Lou attacked the problem with excessively heavy weights, used progressively. He would alternate standing calf raises with seated calf work and put more and more weight on each machine every week. It was not long before Lou's lower legs measured over 20 inches.

The calf muscle along with the forearms, has long been considered a difficult area to build up. This becomes clear especially to those not blessed with genetic potential.

Many blacks do not have the genetics to build a full, diamond-shaped, large calf muscle. Their kind of calf, known as a high calf, is located high up the leg and resembles a tight knot of muscle rather than a fully-rounded, balanced lower leg. It cannot be wholly altered. The muscle itself can be enlarged through regular hard work, but it will not develop lower down on the leg where there are few, if any, cells.

Robby Robinson had this type of high calf, but he overcame the problem via a two-point plan:

1. He worked very hard on building up what calf cells he did possess.

2. He reduced his heavy thigh work so that his thighs and calves now "flow" where they formerly appeared like "drum-sticks" supporting enormous oversized thighs.

Today Robby's legs have a very pleasing appearance, from top to bottom.

Ironically, although many blacks have this frustrating high calf phenomenon, the very best calves in the bodybuilding field belong to blacks. Chris Dickerson, Bertil Fox and Johnny Fuller each have superb lower legs.

Ballet dancers invariably have superb calves, in spite of often possessing small ankles and knees. Of course a ballet dancer often makes the grade *because* he has good-looking legs, as well as for his ability to dance, jump and otherwise perform on stage. Nevertheless, there is sufficient evidence to show that the constant work on the toes via jumps, heel raises, etc., that the ballet performer does several hours every day, helps.

A trick that one British bodybuilder used to bring up his resistant calves and one which you may like to try, is to attach two blocks of wood about 3 to 4 inches thick to the soles of a pair of worn-out sandals (simply bang a few nails through the leather sole into the block beneath). Practice walking on these, taking care to rise high up on the block each step, and alternately lower down completely until your heels touch the ground. Our British bodybuilder, who was a little self-conscious doing this, would drive out to the country after dark and walk a couple of miles on these unique "shoes." Within a four-month period he added 2 inches to his underpinnings and actually won the Mr. Britain title.

"Block shoes" are only supplementary to the basic calf training program, however.

The most proven way of building calves, however, is to follow a system of stretching the calves with several sets of nonapparatus calf raises (concentrating on attaining a maximum stretch, both up and down), combined with three or four regular weekly sessions of very heavy calf raises, using at least 15 reps per set, always with a view to increasing resistance whenever possible.

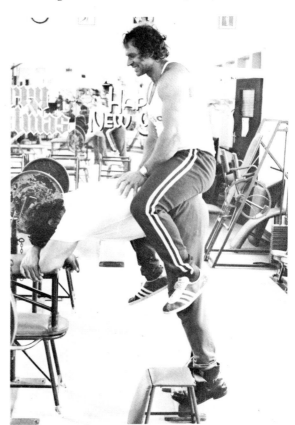

Illus. 183.   Donkey calf raise performed by Reg Park.

Veteran Vince Gironda advises trainers to always work the calves on a 6-inch block (to allow for maximum stretch) covered with a ½-inch layer of glued-on gum rubber padding. Gironda also believes that it is best to do all calf work barefoot to maximize total stretch. It may be observed that most top bodybuilders perform their calf work with rather than without sneakers.

Larry Scott (who does his calf work barefoot) works extensively with the donkey calf raise until the burn becomes almost unbearable. He then bends his knees for a few moments, and rises up on his toes, to allow the flow of blood to run freely, which alleviates the pain, and allows him to continue further calf raises.

Stubborn calves will not react to regular training unless the progressive (weight adding) element is present. Do not make the mistake of thinking that "getting a burn" will build Herculean lower legs. A friend of mine (with 15-inch calves) was explaining to Arnold Schwarzenegger how he performed his calf exercises on a seated leg press machine. "It gives me a real burn," he told "the Oak." Arnold grinned . . . "Listen," he retorted with his thick Austrian accent, "if I lit a match under your backside you would get a burn, but that doesn't mean you'd get bigger!" We all laughed, but Arnold had made his point. Work heavy and hard for maximum calf development.

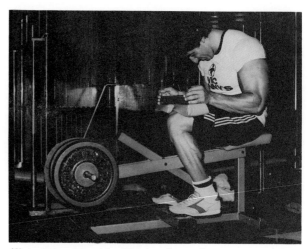

Illus. 185. *Seated calf raise shown by uncrowned Mr. Olympia Dennis Tinerino.*

Donkey Calf Raise

There is no doubt that the "bent-over" position one adopts for the donkey calf raise exercise does something very special for the lower legs. This is a great favorite of Mr. Olympia Frank Zane:

Lean on a bench or table top so that your upper body is comfortably supported parallel to the floor. A training partner sits on your lower back, over the hip area. Rise up and down on your toes, until you cannot perform another rep. Use a 4-inch block under the toes to give greater range to the foot movement. You should always aim to perform at least 20 reps in this exercise.

Standing Calf Raise

It is important that the calf machine you use is capable of loading on heavy weights. The apparatus should either carry a huge stack of weights or else be set up with a leverage benefit so that comparatively small amounts of weight give considerably increased overall load.

Rise up and down on your toes without excessive knee bend and without bouncing at the bottom of the movement.

Seated Calf Raise

This exercise too is performed on a special leverage machine. The principal muscle worked in this movement is the *soleus* rather than the *gastroc-*

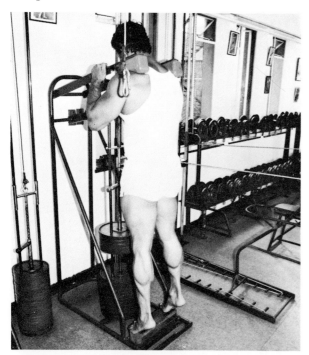

Illus. 184. *Standing calf raise by Reg Park.*

nemius. Perform as many heel raises as you can, concentrating on maximizing total calf stretch with each repetition.

Leg Press Machine Calf Raise

Calf raises may also be performed on the leg press machine. Some of these machines are set at an angle (as in Illus. 186) while others are set up so that the movement is performed lying on the back with legs vertical. Get as much extension as possible with this exercise, pointing the toes as much as possible in the "up" position and lowering them as far as possible in the "down" position.

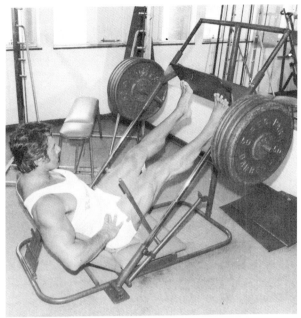

Illus. 186.   Calf raise on leg press machine, demonstrated by Reg Park, multi-Universe winner.

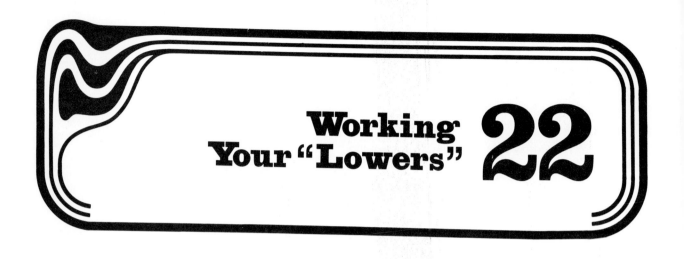

Working Your "Lowers" 22

Like a sculptor or architect, a bodybuilder must always be aware of what he's doing. He must plan for physical balance—perfection if you will—and, more importantly, he must follow through on the plan. There are today literally hundreds of thousands of bodybuilders around. A great many of them build large muscles but still do not quite make the grade in physique contests because they have deviated from a common-sense plan.

You have to work your "lowers" for bodybuilding success. No great champ has ever neglected them. "Lowers" include: (1) lower arms or forearms; (2) lower lats (back); (3) lower legs or calves; (4) lower thighs; (5) lower biceps; (6) lower triceps and (7) lower abdominals.

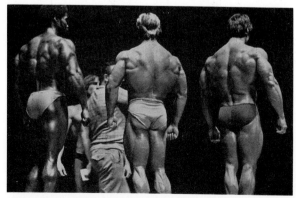

Illus. 187.   Robby, Platz and Padilla show remarkable "lowers" in this Olympia shot.

A winning physique today has more than just muscle thrown onto a frame. It has quality, proportion and "line." It is a finished, completely developed body with no weak points. The seven "lowers" I have listed are all essential to that overall perfect physique.

Forearms

Arnold Schwarzenegger used to neglect his forearms, believing that a small forearm would make his upper arm look even bigger. The biting remarks of his early training buddy Frank Zane finally convinced Arnold to work his forearms extensively. Ultimately Arnold built impressive forearms of great power, superseding perhaps even Zane's own lower arm development. Big forearms only heighten the upper arms. Men noted for their huge forearms include old-timers Chuck Sipes, Dave Draper, Larry Scott and Bill Pearl and among the recent champs, Tim Belknap (Mr. America 1981), Casey Viator, Mike Mentzer, Jusup Wilcosz, Lou Ferrigno and Boyer Coe, all with sensational lower arm development.

Forearms are used in practically every exercise yet unless you are naturally endowed, you have to work them with specific exercises to really get them to grow.

Current favorites described in chapter 15 of this book include wrist curls, reverse wrist curls and reverse curls. Some champs use a special plate loading device in which the grip raises the weight a few inches. Some bodybuilders enjoy using the wrist roller technique for building their forearms. This involves a short bar with a disc tied to the end of a cord. By rotating the bar with your wrists (forearms) the cord "winds" up the weight. The exercise can be torturously effective. Use at least 15 reps in your forearm exercises and do about 8 to 10 sets of overall forearm work each time you train them (at least twice a week).

If you fail to get sufficient forearm stimulation from using "straight sets" you could graduate to the pre-exhaust method of training. A suitable combination of moves would be to alternate sets of wrist curls with close-grip chins or reverse wrist curls with close-grip upright rowing; no resting between sets.

Lower Lats

Depending on your lower lat muscle insertion, you will find it easy or difficult to build the area. The important thing is that no bodybuilder must be without full lower lat development.

The best lower lat exercises are T–bar rowing, the single-arm dumb-bell row and the bent-over barbell row. Make sure in each case that the weight is pulled "low" into the waist and not up to the chest. Many bodybuilders also enjoy the seated cable pulls, again always pulling towards the waist area.

Close-grip chins (hands eight inches apart) attempting to touch the chest to the bar is also a fine movement (if you can do it!) for the lower lats. Some trainers like to use a triangle close-grip attachment so they are able to hold with two hands either side of the chin bar, palms facing inward. The lower lats are brought even more into action.

Calves

Third on our list of "lowers" is the biggest bugaboo of all—calves. If you are lacking in this area you must work hard on calf training, exercising them for at least 8 to 12 sets per workout. Many physiques have failed to impress because of poor or nonexistent calf development, yet many men who have made the most of relatively poor calf development have gone on to win international titles. Lou Ferrigno, Arnold Schwarzenegger and Reg Park all had lower leg "problems" early on in their training but they concentrated work on their calves until they turned the situation around completely. Each did it in more or less the same way, using very heavy

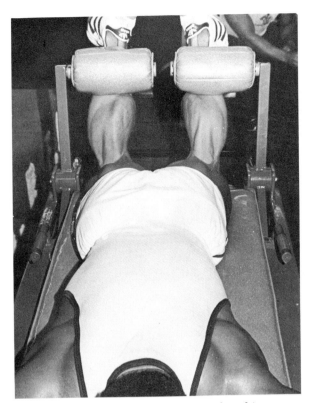

Illus. 188.   Chris Dickerson enjoys working his "lowers" with the thigh-curl machine. His calves are among the greatest.

poundages on the standing calf machine for at least 10 sets of 15 to 25 reps per set.

Men like Chris Dickerson, Mike Mentzer, Johnny Fuller, Steve Reeves, Ken Waller and Casey Viator all have natural calf impressiveness, but for every natural, there are a hundred men who have to train their lower legs extremely hard to keep them in line with the easier-growing thighs. Both Schwarzenegger and Park worked up until they were using over 1,000 pounds on the machine for sets of 20 reps.

Carl Richford, noted bodybuilding authority and writer, states that bodybuilders lacking in calf development should learn to walk properly: "Don't walk flat-footed, or by swinging the leg forward at the knee. Come down on your heel, rolling forward on the foot so your toe is down and heel up. Push forward off your toe, in effect making each step a toe raise. When you go upstairs, do so on your toes, not flat-footed. The same goes for running.

"In calf raises, as in forearms, form and number of exercises are limited by the lack of mobility of the joint. All you can do is go up and down, but the average bodybuilder seems even incapable of doing this right. For gains you must have as full a range of

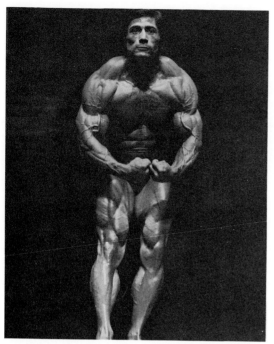

Illus. 189.   Danny Padilla—superbly endowed with full muscular development.

Illus. 190.   Casey Viator—No problem with proportion. He's built from head to toe!

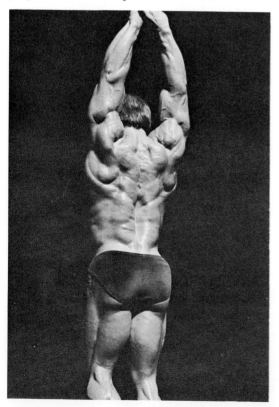

motion as possible, which means going up all the way and down all the way. Stretching down is vitally important and usually neglected. Also abused is standing form, for elementary mechanics shows you the angle is a lever, with the toe one point, the shoulder or hips, wherever the weight is, the other; and the ankle, the fulcrum.

"Therefore you should keep your knees locked, your shoulders straight, and the weight over the foot. Unlock the knees, slouch your back, and have the weight at an awkward point means a waste of the exercise. For this reason I think the donkey toe raise is better to do—you cannot cheat on form so easily. Seated toe raises with the weight across your knees, are also fine as long as you go through a full range of motion. Needless to say, high reps and sets are essential for growth too."

Lower Thighs

Parallel squats are the best overall thigh developing exercise. They build the upper and middle areas more than adequately. In the case of the short-legged individual, the squat will even build the lower thigh, but for the majority of us the lower thigh needs special attention.

What made Steve Reeves so extraordinary? He had great lower thighs. Virtually every other star of his day possessed big bulky upper thighs, but it was Reeves who got all the praise because of his lower thighs. He had an abundance of muscle just above the knee, which made his legs the most eye-catching part of his physique. Reeves built his lower thighs by performing hack lifts (squatting up and down while holding a barbell behind the thighs) and front squats (holding a barbell in front of the neck, elbows raised high). In both instances he supported his heels with a 3-inch wooden block, a ploy to take the action away from the hips, thus avoiding a large rump.

A modern way to quickly build up the lower thighs is to pre-exhaust them, by first doing a set of hack slides (or barbell hack squats or leg extensions) and then following these with a compound movement such as the regular back squat. This is a technique popularized by Mr. Universe, Mike Mentzer, whose thighs are somethin' else!

Fully developed thighs mean fully developed *lower* thighs, cut-to-ribbons-and-built thighs! Anyone can have upper thigh and hip development, but the thing that will make that "V" shape really stand out is the complete development of your lower thighs. It is one of the "secrets" of a championship body.

Lower Biceps

It could be argued that if you have short, high, "balled-up" biceps, there is not a lot you can do to lengthen them. I tend to agree with that statement, but, on the other hand, if you have this kind of biceps development, typified by a large gap between your biceps and elbow joint, it would make sense to aim 90 percent of your biceps exercises specifically at the *lower* regions. It is this emphasis on the weaker lower bi's and the corresponding avoidance of exercises which build the stronger upper bi's that will combine to help your biceps look more balanced.

The first thing to do when going for lower biceps development is to avoid cheating curls. The lower biceps are activated mainly at the start of the curl, as soon as the arm begins to bend. Accordingly your curl should always be started *slowly* from a completely "straight-armed" position.

The king of movements for lower biceps development is the preacher bench curl, when performed at bench angles of 45° or shallower. A steep-angled bench, although ideal for peaking the arms, is not an exercise for building the "lowers".

Make it a habit to perform all chinning exercises and rowing motions (upright and bent-over varieties) in a very strict manner where you always return to the straight-arm position before slowly commencing the next pulling repetition. It is the first few inches of these movements (and the curl) which works the lower biceps. Keep them strict and concentrate mentally on starting each repetition slowly and deliberately, without even the slightest hint of a swing or cheat.

Another lower biceps aid is the thumbs-up dumb-bell curl. Also the reverse grip barbell (or E-Z bar) curl has great application to correcting this problem.

There is a particular beauty in having long, full biceps development. Men like Larry Scott, Steve Reeves, Bertil Fox and Mike Mentzer all have long loping lower bi's which always attracted vociferous praise and admiration. On the other end of the scale men like Clancy Ross, Franco Columbu and Tony Pearson could be described as having something short of lower biceps perfection.

Lower Triceps

Like high biceps, the triceps can also detract from the overall appearance of the physique. If you build them high near the deltoid, the arm seen from the side in the straight position, will appear to taper from the shoulder bulk to a diminishing elbow region, when in fact, aesthetics would have the upper arm muscles holding on to its mass right to the crook of the arm, tucking neatly into the elbow region only to swell again dramatically at the forearm.

If you have too much triceps bulk near the shoulder, *avoid* the lying triceps curl. Perform the single arm triceps extension while in the seated or standing position. Another good lower triceps move is the back press with strands and the standing close grip barbell (or E-Z bar) stretch behind head, holding the elbows as close to the ears as possible. The best lower triceps movement I know is the bent-over dumb-bell extension to the rear, a great favorite of Larry Scott's (torso and upper arm parallel to floor).

Again as with other "difficult" areas, you may use the pre-exhaust principle to blitz the lower tricep. Try alternating (without rest) the close-grip seated triceps stretch with some "combination" parallel bar dips. That should do the trick!

Lower Abdominals

With bodybuilding contests increasing in popularity and with the introduction of substantial money prizes into the sport, the bodybuilder is finding that he has to develop every inch of his body. Whereas in the old days it was quite acceptable if a contestant had only a couple of rows of abdominal muscles to show the judges, today he has to have abs above and below the belt!

In addition to the hanging leg raise which is the best single exercise for the lower abs described in the section on abdominals, another good exercise is the Roman chair sit-up, whereby the body is lowered way down below the hips in each repetition. This is a favorite exercise of Californian Irvin "Zabo" Kozewski who for 35 years has performed this exercise three times a week, training not by counting repetitions but by timing himself by the clock, frequently exercising nonstop for up to 40 minutes at a time. Zabo has won more best abdominal awards than any other man on earth!

All your "lowers" are essential for a pleasingly balanced, prize-winning body. Take a careful look at your body. Remove those rose-tinted spectacles: Develop a critical eye and see if you don't need to work at least some of your "lowers". And do it *now* for it could mean the difference between success and failure.

Principles and Techniques in a Nutshell 23

Weight training, as you may have already discovered, is more complicated than you imagined. In recent years the sport has become far more sophisticated. Modern bodymen are conversant with numerous techniques, principles and advancements that they have found useful to varying degrees.

Here are a few of the more popular and workable systems:

Straight Sets

The straight sets system, for all its simplicity, has possibly produced more muscle for more people than any other method known. Straight sets simply implies that a trainer performs a series of repetitions (a "set") of a particular exercise, pauses for 30 to 90 seconds, and then resumes further sets of the same exercise, allowing for subsequent "rests" between each set. Generally speaking, the number of sets per exercise is between three and five.

Should the exerciser choose to perform another movement for the same body part, it is usual to group the exercises for each body part together. For example, one would group all the chest exercises and together, all the leg exercises, shoulders, biceps, triceps, and so forth.

Straight sets have been used for almost a century but, extensively only after World War II. Virtually every bodybuilder of renown has used the straight-sets technique more than any other.

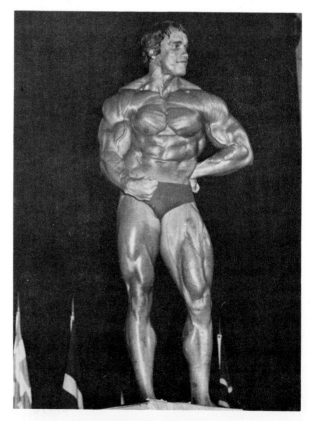

Illus. 191.   Seven-time Mr. Olympia Arnold Schwarzenegger (USA) has used almost every style of training to reach success.

Forced Reps

Although forced reps (sometimes known as "going to full exhaustion") have been practiced since the earliest days of bodybuilding, I first became aware of this technique during the heavy training years of Steve Reeves in the '50s. John Carl Grimek, the only two-time Mr. America, who observed Steve then wrote:

"Watching Steve Reeves train in the old York gym was both educational and inspiring. Steve would perform higher reps than most other stars of the day, and he liked to work his entire body each workout, training three times a week. Often I would see Steve performing an exercise such as the seated dumb-bell curl, where he would curl the weight ten or twelve times, and when the moment came where he was unable to perform another rep, he would kick the weight up with his foot and lower it slowly, thus taking advantage of the negative side of the exercise. At other times he would cheat curl a heavy barbell and lower it as slowly as he could."

Today the forced reps concept has been revived by Michael Mentzer of California. Mike says: "All exercises are divided into two distinct phases. The raising of the weight is called concentric contraction, and the lowering of it, the return to starting position from the point of full contraction to full extension, is called eccentric contraction. It is my opinion that eccentric or *negative* contraction is more productive than the concentric part.

"The negative portion of an exercise allows you to handle even the heaviest weight productively after a muscle has apparently been exhausted. The truth is that even though a trainee may find himself incapable of managing a complete curl on his own, there is still a lot of power left in the muscle that should be exhausted in pursuit of the best results. By allowing a training partner to help him get the weight up, the trainee will discover he is still capable of a few *negative* repetitions . . . which is to say, he can still do three or four more curls, half-curls if you like, by allowing the weight to fall slowly back to the starting position. Of course, he must retain control of the action as the weight comes slowly down. When he is no longer able to control the negative resistance, then the trainee can rest assured the muscle (in this case the biceps) has been fully exhausted by *both* the concentric and the *negative* contractions. Thus you will increase training intensity and force the muscle to cope with the added stress, which will most definitely lead to more positive bodybuilding results."

It should be noted that negative reps are not suited to all. You have to have an exceptional capacity to "take it": Even the hardiest bodybuilders only practice negative reps for some of their exercises some of the time; never all of their exercises all of the time. It would burn you out. Negative reps require more recuperation time and can lead to some mighty sore muscles if you are not used to heavy exercise, so take it easy when first trying this technique.

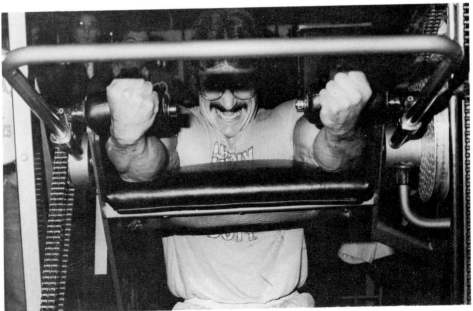

Illus. 192. "Today the forced reps concept has been revived by Michael J. Mentzer."

Heavy Duty

Heavy duty is a name applied to almost any durable product nowadays. In bodybuilding it is the "trade-mark" of Mr. Universe Mike Mentzer.

The method denotes Mentzer's singular philosophy of performing exercises to their "limit" and consequently performing no more than one or two sets. The key word to Mentzer's heavy duty is *intensity*. He achieves high intensity by employing techniques such as forced reps, negative resistance, pre-exhaust and rest-pause. The heavy-duty method has made inroads into almost every champion's training schedule in one way or another. Although it has not been accepted universally by weightmen it is nevertheless giving excellent results to many throughout the world.

Supersets

All muscles pull; they do not really push, but only contract and shorten. The upper arm's biceps muscle contracts and pulls the forearm upwards. The triceps muscle, in back of the arm pulls the arm straight. Bodybuilders, however call them *pulling* and *pushing* muscles.

Pushing exercises include the standing press, supine bench presses, push-ups, triceps extensions and leg presses. *Pulling* exercises refer to upright rows, curls, chins, bent-over rowing and thigh curls.

The idea of *supersets* was to alternate two exercises rapidly without rest—one pulling and one pushing movement. It was common to alternate curls with triceps extensions, but many top bodybuilders would simply alternate two curling movements, two pectoral movements or two triceps movements, not caring whether a particular muscle was being worked against its antagonistic partner (for example, the biceps and triceps). Today, supersets merely refers to the alternation of two exercises in rapid succession.

This type of exercising can jolt the muscles into new growth in weeks, but it is very severe; too much could cause you to grow stale and come to a standstill. Paradoxically, you can break a standstill with a week or two of supersetting your exercises.

Cheating

Also known as "loose" training style, or sloppy form, cheating is the use of the stronger, larger muscles, usually in the legs and back, to assist the performance of an isolation exercise. It is proper to

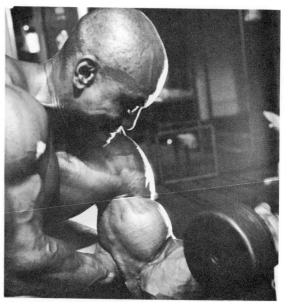

Illus. 193. The superstar of the 60s and 70s was Sergio Oliva. He has used every method including P.H.A., straight sets and the cheating principle.

perform the curl, for example, by standing upright and, starting with arms straight at one's side, beginning to curl the bar up until it is just under the chin. The body should remain upright throughout the lift. This is known as correct, or strict, exercise style. If the legs, hips and back are used to thrust the weight upwards, it is called cheating.

Other common ways of cheating are:

Bending the knees and throwing the weight upward in any type of standing press movement

Leaning back during seated or standing press

Bouncing up and down during squatting movements

Raising the back while doing bent-over rowing

Bouncing the bar on the chest during bench pressing

Allowing the torso to lean back during seated or standing curls

Leaning forward in the lateral raise

Cheating is useful in adding muscle size, but some forms of it, such as bouncing out of a low squat, can be hazardous. It is generally not recommended. The most accepted forms of cheating are the lean-back in the curl and forward leaning at the start of the lateral raise. Not allowed is any form of cheating that either bounces a weight on a vulnerable area or causes unreasonable stress to a joint, such as bouncing squats (knees) or dumb-bell triceps curls (elbows).

Peak Contraction

As the bar begins travelling upwards during the curl, the first part of this lift is easy. As the forearms approach the parallel-to-floor position, the most strenuous point of the exercise, the biceps are at their *peak contraction*. After this point, the movement becomes relatively easy again. The peak contraction principle applies to those few movements in body, arm or leg positions whose hardest parts come at the *conclusion* of the exercise. The crunch sit-up (with legs raised on a bench), thigh curls on a steep incline, upside-down sit-ups from an overhead bar and the bent-over rowing movement probably use this principle most. Like most advanced methods, the peak contraction principle is severe and should be only occasionally included in your exercise routine.

Up and Down the Rack

If you are lucky enough to have your own full set of dumb-bells, ranging from pairs of 5 pounders all the way up to pairs of 90s, 100s or even more, this system works wonders. Most of us don't, though, so it's usually used in the gym.

The name explains the method. Any exercise that you usually do standing up with dumb-bells can be chosen. Start with a light pair and do a given number of repetitions, go up to the next heaviest pair, and so on. When you can no longer perform several repetitions because of the heavier resistance, start *coming down* the rack, using increasingly lighter dumb-bells.

This is an outstanding method of promoting new growth when applied to exercises like standing dumb-bell presses, dumb-bell curls or lateral raises, and the pump is unsurpassed.

Compound Training

Compound training, or "giant" sets, is an advanced muscle building technique. If you wanted to work the deltoids, a compound set would involve doing three or four shoulder exercises, one after the other, with minimal rest between exercises. The compound-training principle applied to the shoulders would consist of:

Press behind neck	10 reps
Seated dumb-bell presses	10 reps
Upright rowing	10 reps
Standing lateral raise	10 reps
Short Rest	

Repeat the entire routine twice more for a total of three sets.

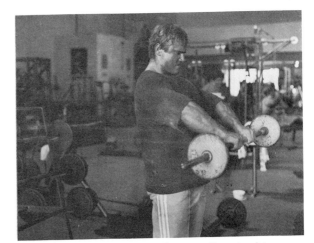

Illus. 194.   Tom Platz, seen here performing his special "hold-out" upright rows is a product of scientific weight training. His workouts are a sight to believe!

Illus. 195.   Al Beckle's secret is conditioning. He does not miss workouts. Ever!

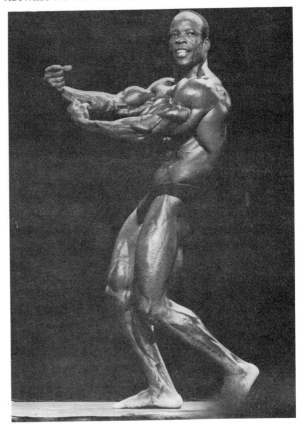

Pre-Exhaust

The *pre-exhaust* system is based on attacking a specific muscle with a carefully chosen isolation exercise, followed immediately by a combination movement.

Take the pecs. The triceps involved in many of the recognized chest exercises are, in most people, the weakest link. In dips, bench presses, or incline presses, the triceps are worked hard but the pectorals only moderately, so the triceps grow more rapidly than the chest. If you already have a big chest, it doesn't matter, but if you want to develop your pecs, here's where the pre-exhaust method will help.

To get around the triceps, isolate the pecs first by using an exercise where the triceps are not directly involved, like the dumb-bell flyes. Carrying the exercise to the point of failure, go right to a second exercise, such as the incline press or bench press.

After the presses, the triceps will temporarily be stronger than the pectorals, which are in a state of near exhaustion from the first isolation exercise. You need not be limited by the "weak link" triceps.

The Pre-Exhaust Schedule

SHOULDERS:

Isolation Movement
Lateral Raise with dumb-bells

Combination Movement
Press Behind Neck *or* Upright Rowing

CHEST:

Isolation Movement
Low Incline Flye *or* Cable Cross-Over

Combination Movement
Medium Grip Bench Press *or* Incline Bench Press

THIGHS:

Isolation Movement
Thigh Extension

Combination Movement
Leg Press *or* Squats

BACK:

Isolation Movement
Lat Shrugs on parallel bars keeping arms straight throughout. Try to touch ears with shoulders

Combination Movement
T–Bar Rowing or Bent-Over Rows to waist

ABDOMINALS:

Isolation Movement
Crunches

Combination Movement
Hanging Leg Raise

CALVES:

Isolation Movement
Calf Raise

Combination Movement
Rope Jumping

BICEPS:

Isolation Movement
Scott Preacher Bench Curls

Combination Movement
Narrow Undergrip Chins

TRICEPS:

Isolation Movement
Triceps Pressdowns on lat machine *or* one-arm Triceps Stretch

Combination Movement
Narrow Grip Bench Press (hands 2 inches apart)

FOREARMS:

Isolation Movement
Reverse Wrist Curls

Combination Movement
Reverse Curls

If you wish to "split" this routine so that you train four or five times a week working only half the schedule at one time, it is suggested that you work legs, back and biceps one day, and chest, shoulders, triceps and forearms on alternate days. The waist can be worked every day.

The amount of sets and reps you do is entirely up to you. Those new to pre-exhaust should perhaps hold their sets down to two. As your condition improves you may perform up to 5 sets of each exercise but no more. Reps should average around 10. Some trainers will get best results doing sets of 8 whereas others may get more from utilizing a scheme of 12 reps or even more.

Wankers Routine

Wankers is a variety of low-intensity training. Possibly a reaction to the hard-pushing heavy-duty principle, the Wankers routine is not exactly for the faint-hearted, either. Wankers uses about three exercises per body part with 8 to 15 reps per set, and 5 sets per exercise. The progressive factor is still important. You must increase poundages once you are used to the system, but never at the expense of style or through excessive strain.

Growth is achieved by getting in plenty of sets and reps. Accordingly, the Wankers routine often is a wonderful substitute for more strenuous systems, a change is as good as a rest.

Unlike the heavy duty principle, the Wankers routine is not a super-fast way to "rope-sized" tendons and "rip cord" strength, but is a good way to pump up your muscle cells to maximum size. Because your repetitions are fairly high the weights used will be only moderate, rather than exessively heavy. There should, however, be a concerted effort to lessen the rest period between sets and increase the speed of your repetitions while maintaining perfectly strict style. No cheating is permitted with the Wankers routine.

Free-Style Training

Steve Reeves, Dave Draper and Charlie Smith have all made excellent gains using the free-style training method.

Free-style training is just what it implies: training all body parts in one workout, although some areas may get more of a workout on particular days. According to its main proponent, Dave Draper, "Free-style training is practiced according to how you feel on any given day. It is fantastic for building strength and cardiovascular efficiency." Draper continues, "I use many compound movements and train six days a week, so I don't think this form of training will suit everybody. I suggest most bodybuilders break into it gradually. Perhaps a routine that is 75 percent conventional and 25 percent free style will be ideal at first."

In free-style training you usually group your body part exercises together, but you are not restricted as to the number of reps, sets or exercises you do. That is left up to basic instinct. You may, for example, want to blitz your chest and take it easy on the legs in one workout. Another time, because you feel *ready* for it, your legs will be given the "third degree."

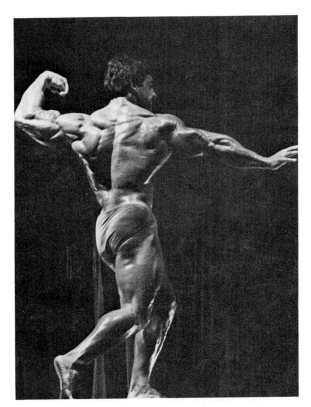

Illus. 196.   Bob Kennedy invented the pre-exhaust method, but Mike Mentzer is probably its greatest pioneer and promoter.

Advanced free-style training does provide for working the entire body every other day or splitting the workout into two halves and training six days a week.

The Triple Drop

This is a pretty old technique enjoying a revival in the weight-training field. Triple dropping is best described as the performance of 3 sets in one, reducing the weight each set. As an example, if you are doing the curl exercise, pick up a set of dumb-bells that would allow you to perform say, 6 reps. Let's assume you chose a pair of 50 pounders. Now as part of the triple-drop technique, you should also take a pair of 40 pounders and also a pair of 30 pounders.

Before commencing your triple drop set you should *always warm up*. It is suggested you use a moderately heavy pair of dumb-bells and perform about 10 reps. This is an absolute *must* and *should not under any circumstances be skipped*, since triple dropping is a very arduous form of exercise and you would not want to tear any muscles.

After the warm-up, take a brief rest and pick up your 50 pounders. The first part of your triple drop is underway.

With perfect exercise style, go all out to get a good 6 hard reps. This is not a warm-up, so you must find yourself near to complete failure by your sixth rep. When you cannot get another rep, place the two 50 pounders on the floor and then without any rest, pick up the two 40 pounders and try your very best to get another 6 reps. After about your second or third rep your biceps will feel as though they are on fire, but this is only a build up of lactic acid inside the muscle.

Although your biceps will be very pumped up causing a painful and burning sensation deep down inside the muscle, you can, with willpower and determination, continue to your sixth rep because *the weight has been reduced.*

After your second set of 6 reps, place the dumb-bells on the floor and pick up the 30 pounders. Although the dumb-bells are very light, you will find it very, very difficult, the first time you do it, to complete another 6 reps.

When you have done as many reps as you possibly can, place the dumb-bells on the floor and your first *triple drop* set is over!

APPLYING TRIPLE DROPPING TO YOUR WORKOUTS

You would be very wise for the first two weeks to do only one of these triple drop sets. This is a very severe form of training which should not be taken to extremes at any time. After two weeks you may find two such triple drop sets are best.

It is probably unwise to triple drop your whole body at each workout. It is far better to just apply the triple-drop method to the one or two body parts you want to grow faster.

Nubret Pro-Rep Method

Serge Nubret of France has a unique way of training. At one time he trained very heavily and could curl over 240 pounds and bench press 500. Today he exercises using a singular, seldom-practiced principle. Nubret introduces progression into his training, not by constantly pushing the poundages higher and higher, but by pushing his rep count up. Actually it is a double progression since he also tries to "race the clock."

For example, if it took 45 minutes to do 30 sets of an exercise one day, the next day Nubret will try to squeeze out 31 or 32 sets in the same length of time. He often wills himself to beat his rep record of

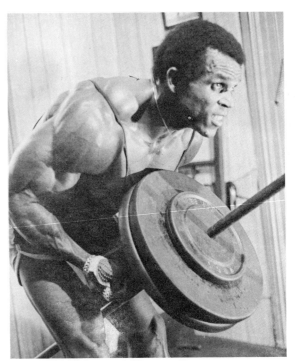

Illus. 197.   France's Serge Nubret pushes his rep count up to give him a unique progression.

the prior set. Using the seated dumb-bell curl, Serge may start off by doing a set of 10 reps with a 45-pound dumb-bell, and in his second set will do 11 reps, his third set 12 reps and so on, all with the same weight. The secret of Nubret's method lies in his ability to "feel" an exercise by pure concentration on the movement he is doing at the time.

Rest Pause

This method has been used since the invention of barbells. Rest pause is not a system to be followed all the time, but it does permit one to greatly increase tendon and muscle strength and add to overall size in a few weeks.

It's a simple idea. After warming up for a particular exercise, you load up the barbell sufficiently to allow just one repetition. Assume you are bench pressing: Press out one difficult rep and replace the bar on the stands. Allow 10 to 20 seconds to elapse and perform another repetition. After a similar brief rest perform yet another rep—and so on. Each time you allow the body to partially recuperate. It's possible that you may have to reduce the weight slightly to attain 6 or 8 reps as the reps mount up.

Rest pause owes its resurgence of popularity to Mike Mentzer, who uses it in his own rugged training program.

Peripheral Heart Action Training

During the 1960s a relatively new form of weight training gained prominence. It appealed to many men in the bodybuilding field because it alleviated the boredom that can come from repeating set after set of the same exercise, contributed to overall heart and lung fitness and speeded up workouts so less time was spent in the gym.

The method known as P.H.A. (Peripheral Heart Action) calls for the performance of one exercise for each main body part with a minimum of rest for four to six different areas. The main feature is that in going from one exercise to another, you select movements which work totally unrelated areas. One would *not*, for example, perform a bench press, then a standing press, followed by dips and arm movements.

A typical P.H.A. series runs through the whole body, jumping from one extremity to another, such as from Press Behind Neck to Front Squat to Barbell Curl to Calf Raise.

In this way the blood does not become congested in one area. The pump as we know it does not exist with P.H.A. Growth still takes place, but truth to tell, it may not be as effective in creating giant muscles as other more forceful methods. But P.H.A. is a *healthy* way to train. It incorporates progressive resistance (you add weight when you can). It utilizes time to advantage since there is no need for rest periods of any length because you are not waiting for a muscle area to partially recover before working it again.

P.H.A. was first popularized nationally, then internationally by the physical education director of the Chicago Y.M.C.A., Bob Gadja. Bob was a total believer in this method of progressive resistance exercise and even had the current world physique phenomenon Sergio Oliva using his methods. In fact the whole bodybuilding world took to P.H.A. after Peary Rader first publicized it in *Iron Man* magazine. Peary liked the method because it had a sane ring to it. He believes that constant pumping of set after set of one exercise is detrimental to the system.

Virtually all the bodybuilding periodicals of the day picked up on it. Most of the champions gave the method a try and some enjoyed great success. It appealed especially to the older trainers who had ambitions beyond mere physical development. It promoted health and well-being—with less injury— and dovetailed neatly with athletic training. A further advantage of the P.H.A. system of training is that the evidence appears to show that recuperation from such training is significantly faster than other "pumping-type" methods. Somehow the waste products in the blood are cleared more rapidly.

The general procedure in setting up a P.H.A. routine is to select four or six exercises for totally different body parts and place them into "cycles." The entire routine would then consist of two, three or four cycles of four to six exercises each cycle.

When you start your "cycle" you first perform exercise number one, then exercise number two, three, and so on. At the end of the first "cycle" you are permitted a short two-minute rest, after which you start at the beginning of that same cycle again.

DURATION OF ROUTINES

IMPORTANT:

Beginners to physical culture should perform only one or two rotations of each "cycle."

Intermediates can perform three rotations of each "cycle."

Advanced may perform up to five rotations of each "cycle."

SOME SUGGESTED ROUTINES

Beginners: (Perform *one or two* rotations of each cycle *only*.)

Cycle One

Bench Press	10 reps
Barbell Curl	10 reps
Squat	12 reps
Seated Press Behind Neck	12 reps

Cycle Two

Bent-Over Rowing	10 reps
Calf Raise (Standing)	10 reps
Incline Sit-ups	20 reps
Straight-Arm Pullover	12 reps
Triceps Stretch (Lying)	10 reps

Intermediates: (Perform 3 rotations of each cycle)

Cycle One

Press Behind Neck	8 reps
Squat	10 reps
Chin Behind Neck	12 reps
Bench Press	8 reps

Cycle Two

Thigh Extension	12 reps
Hanging-Leg Raise	20 reps
Calf Raise	20 reps
Barbell Curl	8 reps

Cycle Three

Incline Flying	10 reps
Thigh Curls	15 reps
Roman Chair Sit-ups	20 reps
Triceps Stretch (Lying)	10 reps

Advanced: (Perform 3 to 5 rotations)

Cycle One

Standing Two-Arm Dumb-bell Press	6 reps
Chin Behind Neck	12 reps
Front Squat (feet on 3-inch block)	10 reps
Wide-Grip Bench Press	8 reps

Cycle Two

Roman Chair Sit-ups	25 reps
Calf Raise	20 reps
Bent-Over Rowing	10 reps
Incline Bent-Arm Flyes	10 reps

Cycle Three

Incline Leg Raise	20 reps
Barbell Curl	10 reps
Donkey Calf Raise	25 reps
Standing Triceps Stretch	10 reps

Cycle Four

Thigh Extensions	12 reps
Incline Dumb-bell Curl	10 reps
Standing Lateral Raise	10 reps
Lying Triceps Stretch	10 reps

Note: Only when you have performed the set number of rotations for your first cycle do you move on to your second cycle. And so on.

Bodybuilding for Women 24

Bodybuilding for women? Why not? Men have monopolized so many sports activities, including pumping iron, for so long that women have felt almost guilty about participating.

Bodybuilding is no longer for men alone. Women weight trainers are now well and truly established. There have, of course, always *been* women bodybuilders. *Strength and Health* and *Iron Man* magazines have been running regular features on women bodybuilders for years, but it took the advent of Lisa Lyon to catapult the sport to new heights. Her original publicity photos showing unusual feminine muscularity somewhat shocked the bodybuilding world. Most men and women were against the "new breed" look and thought Lisa Lyon's muscles were *too* defined. She didn't have large muscles, but somehow her appearance drew a great deal of adverse reaction. She was regarded, at first, as a bodybuilding curiosity. But Lisa Lyon persevered and gradually people started to admire what she had done with her body. Appreciation for Lisa mounted when subsequent photos showed her looking delightfully feminine.

Like Arnold Schwarzenegger before her, Lisa could lay on the baby oil and turn up a mighty "most muscular" pose, even showing a degree of separation or vascularity, while later easily becoming the focus of attention at a party as the most attractive and intelligent woman in the room.

In just a few years, modern bodybuilding for women has established itself, and now has hundreds of thousands of followers around the globe.

Bodybuilding is really *reshaping* the body. Many overweight women and men who take up bodybuilding find that for them it is *body reducing*. Women's training usually entails the use of weights to firm, reduce, build and shape a strong, healthy body of firm, svelte muscle tissue that is outrageously feminine, curvy and attractive.

JANINE AT NYSMA CONVENTION '93

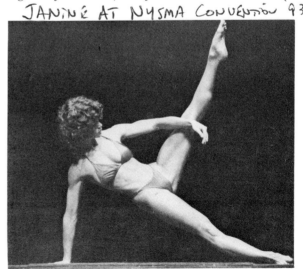

Illus. 198.   Lisa Lyon, who started the new breed of women bodybuilders.

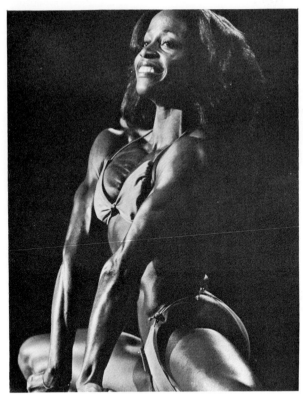

Illus. 199.   Superchamp Carla Dunlap.

The beauty of weights is that you can *tailor* the resistance to your condition. If you are painfully thin and weak, you can start by using extremely light weights so that you ease yourself into condition as the weeks go by. As you get stronger and fill out, you will be able to add a little more weight to the bar. Gradually you will bring yourself up to the kind of shape and condition you've always wanted.

Larger or more athletic women may be able to start with slightly heavier weights, but even so, as a beginner to weight training, you should be prepared to start out "light." There is little sense trying to see how much you can lift when you first get into bodybuilding. This can lead to pulled muscles or minor strains, and ultimately, missed workouts, dejection and confusion.

Remember *you* are in charge of the weights. *You* are using them as tools to sculpt *your* body to physical perfection. The moment you start trying to lift huge barbells that prove too much for your present strength, you have lost control. The weight is boss instead of you.

Once "into" training, a woman can train as hard as a man. In fact Vince Gironda observed at his gym in North Hollywood that women often train *harder* than men. "They're wonderful!" Vince exclaimed, "I

enjoy them because they show the men what it's all about. They have a higher pain threshold, train stricter, harder and are better posers."

Actually women can train using the same exercises as men do. But because they are not aiming for maximum size as are the men, they need not perform a huge amount of sets to fully pump the muscles. Three sets per exercise is usually sufficient.

Bear in mind that your food intake controls both your muscle size and fat content. You can reduce overall size by cutting calories. First the fat will go, then the muscle size itself will diminish if calories are greatly limited. Alternately, muscle size will increase (if you are training hard) when food intake is increased, and naturally a regular oversupply of calories will result in fat accumulation, which is seldom if ever desirable.

Some women bodybuilders could be said to overdo the degree of muscularity they achieve. At a certain point, if all fat reserves are depleted, the woman bodybuilder will cease to have normal periods (they may stop altogether) and the bust area will reduce significantly. Low fat levels at time of competition are advantageous; however, it is not a good idea to aim for body fat levels below eight percent. Although some men have reported getting their body fat levels as low as 2.4 percent, women constitutionally have a higher fat percentage than men and should not aim to equal the levels obtained by their male counterparts.

Never be tempted to take any fat-reducing drugs such as thyroid or amphetamines. They will put you in the hospital faster than anything and possibly give *permanent* side effects.

Criteria for women's posing and contest requirements are still being worked out. Women's bodybuilding is so young a sport that the rules and regulations are still evolving. Doris Barrilleaux from Florida, who was a bodybuilder 20 years before the current explosion in popularity, has been responsible for much of the progress made in the field. Her SPA (Super Physique Association) newsletter has promoted the women's cause a great deal.

Your first workout is important in more ways than one. Since weight training is the most concentrated form of exercise known, I can't stress too strongly that your first few workouts should be performed with very light resistance. Unless you are naturally strong, well-conditioned and superbly fit right now, use *only* the bar for your first workout. Later as you gain strength, you will add some discs to increase resistance.

Sets and Reps

To recap, "reps" (repetitions) are the number of times you perform a particular exercise. If you lift a weight up and down 10 times, that is known as 10 repetitions.

A "set" is one *group of repetitions*. As an example, if you did 10 squats, that is known as *1* set of *10* reps, (usually written 1 × 10). If you do another group (set) of squats, this is known as 2 sets of 10 reps (written 2 × 10).

Beginners should do *only 1 set* per exercise. In two weeks this can be increased to *2* sets per exercise. In four weeks one can graduate to *3* sets. There is seldom any need to perform more than 3 sets of any exercise.

Repetitions are most effective in the 8 to 12 range. Some women will feel they get more from fewer repetitions (6 to 8) while others may prefer performing more (15 to 20). For those completely in the dark about how many repetitions to do, we advise 10.

Exercise Performance

When you lift a weight, the movement should always be smooth and rhythmic. There is no value in struggling with the barbell, leaning backwards to "hoist" it overhead, or bending your knees to jerk it into position. Fluid movement, exercise without strain, is what is needed. Try to raise the weight rhythmically at the same speed that you lower it: up-down, up-down.

Another "must": whenever you lift, be sure you perform the exercise through its entire range of movement: whenever you bend your arms during an arm, shoulder or chest exercise, make sure your arms are always straightened (locked-out) during each repetition. With leg exercises, lock-out on each extension. In this way you will always involve your muscles to their fullest and ensure total flexibility.

Breathing

Proper breathing during your exercise is important. Try to breathe between repetitions. Usually a gulp of air is taken just before the *hardest* part of a movement, and released just as the repetition is *completed*. Try not to hold your breath for any length of time while training. Except in a few non-strenuous movements one should breathe once with each repetition; a quick gulp of air through the mouth, exhaling through pursed lips. Unlike calisthenics, one should *not* breathe through the nose during weight-training exercise.

Rest Periods

After each set of exercises you should take a rest. Either take a brief walk around your exercise area or simply stand still. Sitting down is permissible, but not particularly recommended. In the early stages of training, rest for two minutes between sets of exercises. As you gain strength and stamina, try to reduce your rest period. Aim ultimately to rest only one minute between sets. As a general guide, you should rest long enough for your breathing rate to return to normal.

Concentration

Few things help you more than concentration. Keep your mind on your exercises and results will come quickly. When you are exercising, you should watch yourself in a mirror to keep an eye on your form and control. With practice you can learn to shut out distraction. Don't carry on a running conversation while training. Keep your mind on what you are doing. You will ultimately be in a world of your own during the time you devote to each set. If a bomb went off behind your back, you should hardly notice it.

When to Increase the Weight

Beginners often puzzle over when to increase the weight resistance. Add more weight when the resistance you are using feels too light. Weight training should be pleasurable. You will continually have to increase the resistance as you get stronger, but *not* to the extent of making each exercise an all-out superhuman effort. Train, don't strain. When you can easily do 4 or 5 more repetitions than you have planned for a particular movement, that is the time to increase the resistance. You seldom will need to add more than a couple of 2½-pound discs at a time.

Barbell Collars

Don't train without making sure that your weights are secure. Always use collars tightly fastened onto all barbells and dumb-bells. The last thing you want is a 5-pound disc slipping from the bar onto your big toe.

How Long Should a Workout Be?

Workouts vary in length from one person to another. At first, while you are getting used to performing each exercise, your workout will be longer, maybe 30 minutes or so. Soon you will be able to cut it down to 15 minutes, maybe less. If you really "get into" weights and have a yearning to reach a peak for a beauty contest, or even a specific photo session, then you may want to add a few extra movements which inevitably increase your workout time. However, don't make the common mistake of thinking that more exercises or more sets will necessarily increase the effectiveness of your training. Each person has a different tolerance for weights. What one woman will find only adequate, another will find too demanding. You must not overwork to the point that you feel overtired and drained the next day. Too much exercise is worse than none. If you overtrain you will become listless and bored—and probably end up wanting to forget the whole thing.

Exercises for Beginners

Every workout should begin with a general warm-up period. This can take the form of a two-minute run, four minutes on an exercise bicycle, or a minute spent skipping or running in place. The choice is yours, but don't neglect it. Not only does a warm-up prepare your muscles for their workout, but it will also make you *feel* like training. It is also important to include the stretches described in the "Warming Up" chapter of this book.

I have selected 20 exercises to show you the basics of weight training. To reiterate, a beginner should select only one exercise per body part and perform this 1 set only, using only a light-to-moderate weight to start with. You can always add extra discs as your muscles get used to the exercises.

As you advance, you can perform 2 or even 3 sets of each exercise, depending on your age, personal endurance and recuperative level. Ultimately you may even want to add a second exercise for some of your "weaker" body parts. Remember though, weight training is an extremely concentrated form of exercise and more is not necessarily *better*. It is far preferable to undertrain than to overtrain. I wish you great success!

Seated Dumb-bell Press
(Shoulders and Arms)
(Illus. 200, 201)

Hold a pair of light dumb-bells, 5 to 10 pounds to start, at the shoulders while sitting upright on the end of an exercise bench. (Illus. 200) Press the dumb-bells together to the arms-straight-overhead position and repeat. Breathe in just prior to pressing upwards. Exhale as the arms straighten.

With the use of dumb-bells, each arm is disciplined to work independently. The art of balancing both dumb-bells simultaneously may seem difficult at first, but after a few workouts there will be no problem. If you perform this exercise with the elbows held back most of the work is done by the side deltoids. Perform it with the elbows pointing forward and you will bring the frontal deltoids into play. Do 8 to 12 reps.

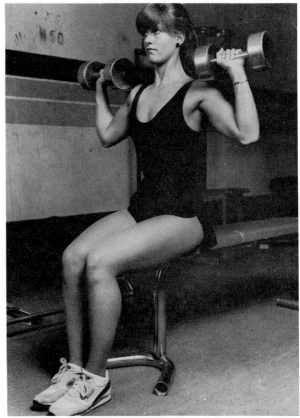

Illus. 200. Seated dumb-bell press (start).

See later in book for "How To Marry a Dumb-bell"

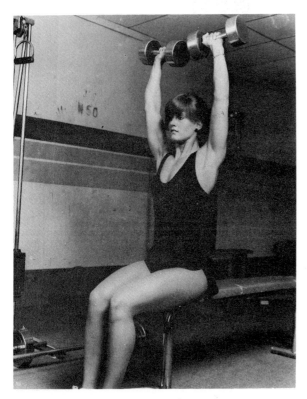

Illus. 201.   Seated dumb-bell press (finish).

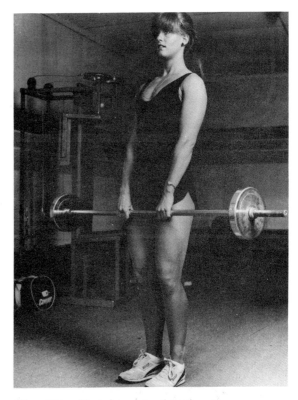

Illus. 202.   Upright rowing (start).

Upright Rowing (Shoulders and Arms)
(Illus. 202, 203)

Hold a barbell at arm's length as shown in Illus. 202, hands about 8 inches apart. Raise the barbell upwards, keeping elbows as high as possible throughout the movement. Lower under control and repeat. Breathe in before starting to raise the weight; exhale as the bar is lowered. Start with about a 20- to 25-pound barbell.

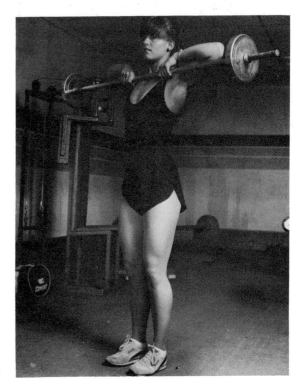

Illus. 203..   Upright rowing (finish).

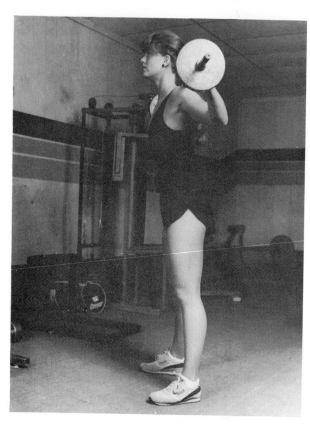

Illus. 204. Start of squat.

Squat (**Thighs**)
(Illus. 204, 205)

The regular barbell squat is like the free-standing squat with the addition of a loaded barbell across the back of your shoulders. If you are very underweight you may want to wrap a towel around the bar where it rests on the upper back to prevent chafing your skin. It is important to keep your head up and your back flat during the entire movement. Starting poundages vary from 30 to 50 pounds, depending on your present strength and condition. Many women bodybuilders are able to squat with double their body weight.

Lower slowly into the squat position keeping the thighs parallel to the floor. Rise slowly to the original upright stance (Illus. 204). At no time should you drop down into a squat and bounce up again. The weight must be under control at all times. Start with about 20 to 30 pounds.

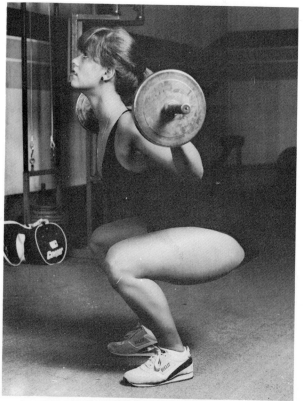

Illus. 205. Finish of squat.

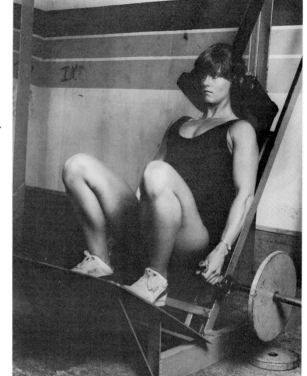

Illus. 206.   Hack slide squats (start).

Hack Slide Squats (**Thighs and Hips**)
(Illus. 206, 207)

You need a hack slide apparatus for this excellent exercise. Start as shown in Illus. 206. Lower into the squat position and immediately rise up. Use only a light weight at first until your body gets used to the movement. Perform 15 to 20 repetitions. Breathe in just before dipping down, exhale as the legs straighten.

Illus. 207.   Hack slide squats (finish).

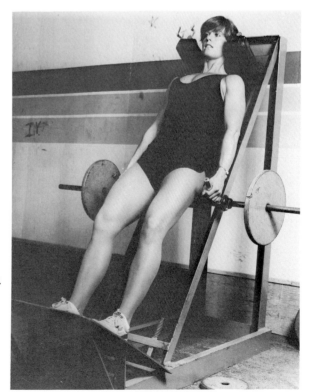

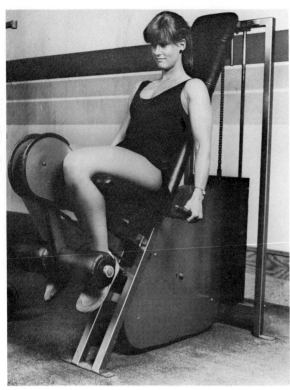

Illus. 208.   Thigh extensions (start).

Thigh Extensions (Upper Legs)
(Illus. 208, 209)

This exercise is done on a special apparatus called a thigh-extension machine. A somewhat watered-down version can be done using a table (or high bench) and a pair of iron boots. Using resistance that is comfortable (about 20 pounds), start in the position shown in Illus. 208 and progress to the legs-straight attitude (Illus. 209). Results from this exercise are more often seen in increased definition and shape rather than size. Try anything from 10 to 15 reps, start the "kick" slowly and do not develop a sloppy swinging-*cum*-bounce style.

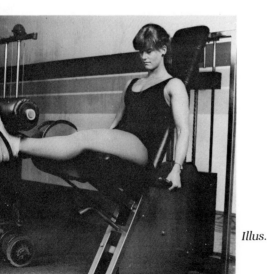

Illus. 209.   Thigh extensions (finish).

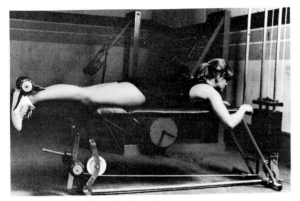

Illus. 210.   Thigh curls (start).

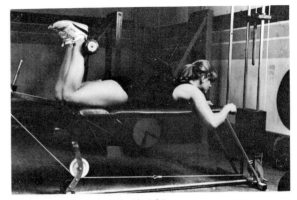

Illus. 211.   Thigh curls (finish).

Thigh Curls (Leg Biceps)
(Illus. 210, 211)

Again using the thigh-extension machine but this time lying on your front, work the thigh biceps through its complete range. Raise the weight from legs-straight to legs-curled position. Try 12 to 15 reps with 10 to 20 pounds on the apparatus. Inhale as you feel necessary.

Bench Press (Chest and Arms)
(Illus. 212, 213)

It doesn't take a genius to see that the bench-press movement is in fact an upside-down floor dip. But it is superior as a chest-building exercise because you do not have to hold your body straight nor do you have to balance to the same extent. The most important advantage is that you can add small amounts of weight to the bar on a regular basis. Before you know it you'll be handling respectable poundage in this exercise. Start with 20 to 40 pounds, and be prepared to handle 100 pounds or more within your first year of training. Inhale as you lower the weight, exhale as it goes up. (Imagine you are blowing it up.) Most people lower the weight to the nipple area, but those who wish to build "higher" pectorals may lower the bar to the upper chest. Under no circumstances allow the weight to bounce from the sternum (chest bone) as this could damage the delicate nerve center located beneath it.

When bench-pressing, grip so that the forearms are vertical when the bar is resting on the chest. Push the weight up to arm's length as shown in Illus. 213. Do not allow the weight to drop, but rather lower it with control to the original position. Perform between 10 to 15 reps.

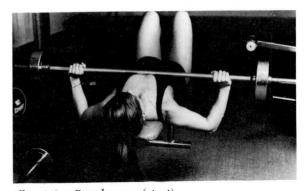

Illus. 212.   Bench press (start).

Illus. 213.   Bench press (finish).

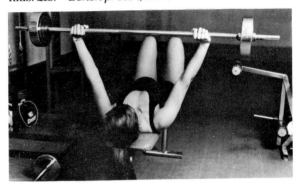

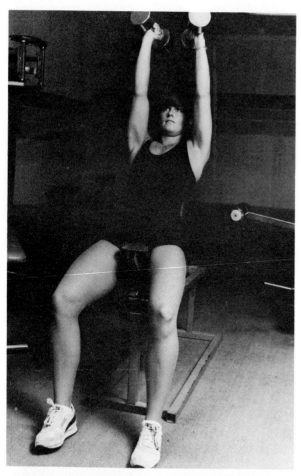

Illus. 214. Incline flyes (start).

Incline Flyes (Upper Chest)
(Illus. 214, 215)

Start with 10- to 15-pound dumb-bells held in the position shown in Illus. 214. Arms are slightly bent throughout the exercise to keep strain off the elbow region. Lower the weights to the position shown in Illus. 215 and return to original position. This exercise mainly builds the pectoral area, especially the outer pecs. Do 10 to 12 reps. As in the bench press, it is a good idea to breathe deeply during the exercise (inhale on the way down, exhale on the way up). This has the long-range effect of aiding rib-cage development.

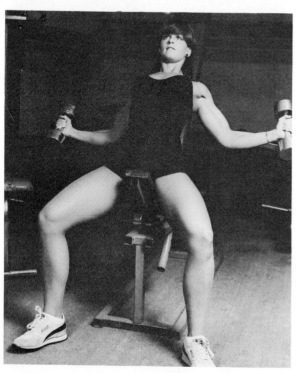

Illus. 215. Incline flyes (finish).

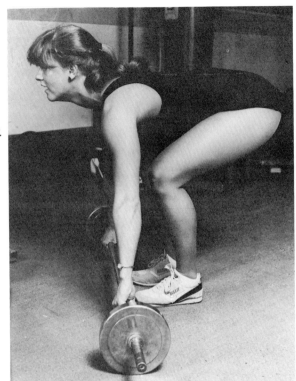

Illus. 216.   Bent-over rows (start).

Bent-Over Rows (Upper Back and Arms)
(Illus. 216, 217)

Set the body into the position shown in Illus. 216, keeping the back flat and the knees slightly bent. Holding a barbell with an overgrip as shown, take a grip width a little wider than shoulder-width. The second part of the movement involves pulling the barbell to the chest. (Begin with about 20 to 30 pounds.) Inhale before lifting, exhale as the weight is lowered. The movement works the entire upper-back and lat area. Do 8 to 12 repetitions.

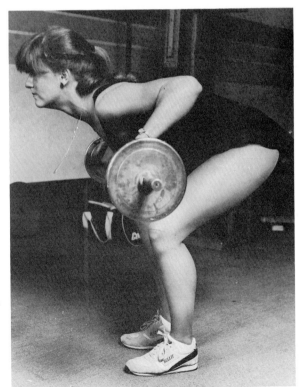

Illus. 217.   Bent-over rows (finish).

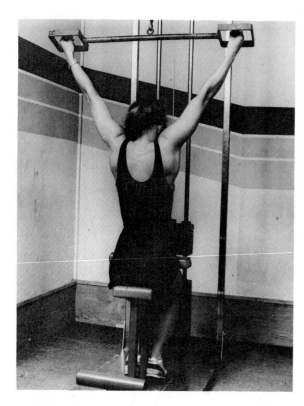

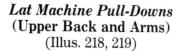

Illus. 218.   Lat machine pull-downs (start).

Lat Machine Pull-Downs
(Upper Back and Arms)
(Illus. 218, 219)

Hold an overhead lat bar using a fairly wide grip. Start with the arms straight and pull the bar down to behind the neck. Return and repeat. Breathe in just before pulling down and release the air slowly as the arms straighten again. Use enough weight to allow for 12 to 15 repetitions without undue strain.

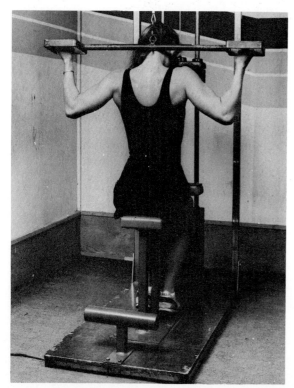

Illus. 219.   Lat machine pull-downs (finish).

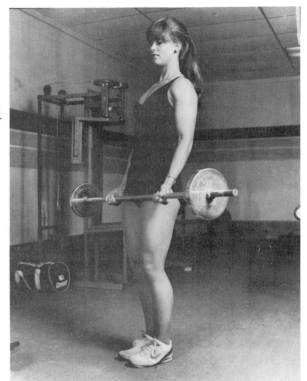

Illus. 220.   Barbell curls (start).

Barbell Curls (**Upper Arms**)
(Illus. 220, 221)

Stand with legs comfortably apart, holding a barbell loaded to about 20 to 30 pounds. Your grip should be about shoulder-width or perhaps slightly wider (Illus. 220). Without leaning back, take a deep breath and curl the barbell to the shoulders as shown in Illus. 221. Do not bend the knees; try to raise the weight while keeping your elbows fairly close to your body. Exhale as the bar arrives at your shoulder level, lower at the same speed at which you raised it and repeat. Try for 12 repetitions. This is the most basic of all biceps exercises and the best one for shaping up that muscle.

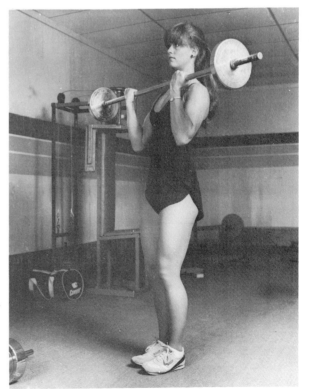

Illus. 221.   Barbell curls (finish).

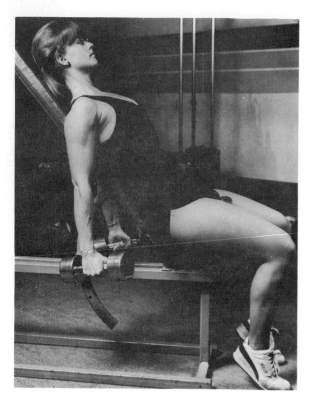

Illus. 222.   Incline dumb-bell curl (start).

Incline Dumb-bell Curl (Upper Arms)
(Illus. 222, 223)

Lying back on a 45°-incline bench, start your curl with straight arms (15-pound dumb-bells are suggested). Inhale as you commence the action, exhale as the arms arrive at the shoulders. Lower at the same speed at which you lifted. Do not permit a "swing" to develop: this takes away from the action. Try 12 reps of this exercise.

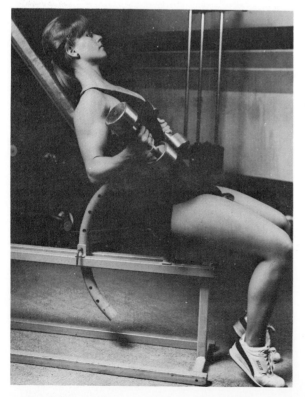

Illus. 223.   Incline dumb-bell curl (finish).

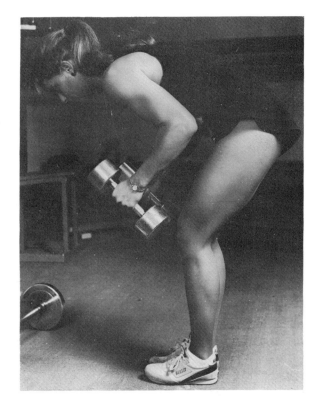

Illus. 224.   Triceps extensions (start).

Triceps Extensions (Upper Arms)
(Illus. 224, 225)

Hold a 5-pound dumb-bell in the bent-over position shown in Illus. 224. The action of the exercise involves the simple extension of the arm (Illus. 225). Breathe as you feel the need; the exercise is not demanding enough to merit deep breathing for every repetition. Do 10 to 15 repetitions.

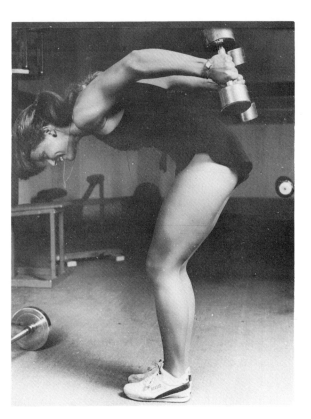

Illus. 225.   Triceps extensions (finish).

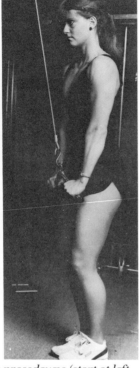

Triceps Pressdowns (Upper Arms)
(Illus. 226, 227)

This exercise can be done only on a special pulley machine. The short bar is held as shown in Illus. 226. Keep the elbows tight into the body and the feet together on the floor. Take a deep breath and push the bar downwards against the up-pulling resistance. Allow the weight to slowly pull the fore-arms up again and repeat the effort 10 to 15 times. Exhale each time as the arms straighten. This is one of the best triceps exercises.

"Good Morning" Exercise (Lower Back)
(Illus. 228, 229)

Start with a light (20-pound) barbell across the upper back as shown in Illus. 228. Keeping the back flat, and holding strongly onto the bar to keep it in position, lower into the second position (Illus. 229). Inhale before going down, exhale as the torso returns to vertical. Try 10 to 20 repetitions. This exercise trains the important lower-lumbar region and has a beneficial effect on the legs, especially the hamstring area at the back of the knees.

Illus. 226 and 227.   Triceps pressdowns (start at left, finish at right).

Illus. 228.   Good-morning exercise (start).

Illus. 229.   Good-morning exercise (finish).

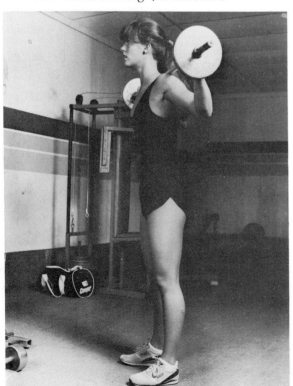

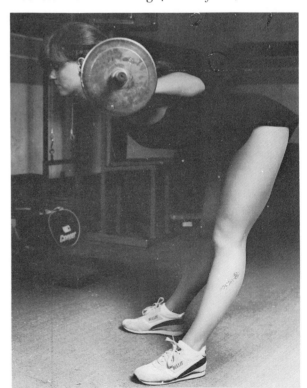

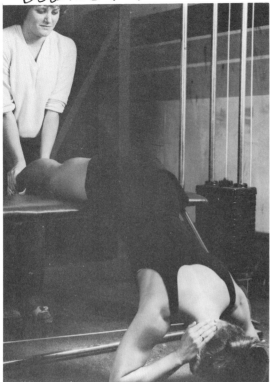

Illus. 230.   Prone hyperextension (start).

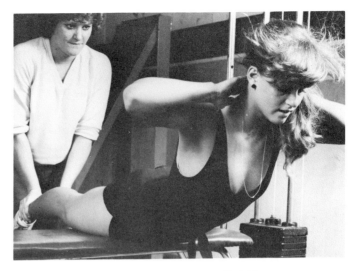

Illus. 231.   Prone hyperextension (finish).

Prone Hyperextension (Lower Back)
(Illus. 230, 231)

Lie face down across an exercise bench. Have a partner hold your legs in place. Start in position shown in Illus. 230 and rise up into the second position. Lower and repeat. Try to eventually do 15 repetitions. This exercise may also be performed on a special padded bench known as a hyper-extension unit.

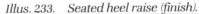

Illus. 232.   Seated heel raise (start).

Illus. 233.   Seated heel raise (finish).

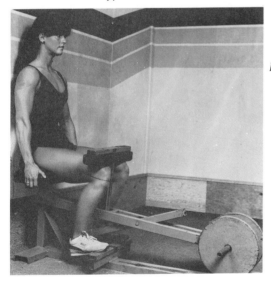

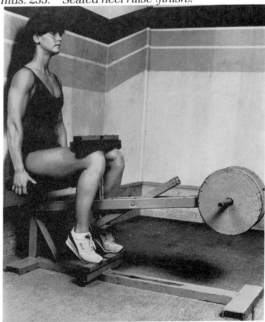

Seated Heel Raise (Calves)
(Illus. 232, 233)

This is an advanced exercise usually performed on a special seated calf-machine. An alternative is to have someone place a heavy barbell across your knees (make sure you have padding). Move up and down, using about 50 pounds of resistance. This exercise builds shape in the *soleus* area of the calf.

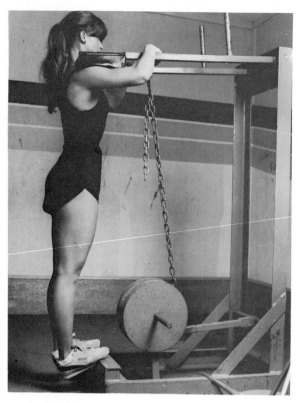

Illus. 234.   Calf raise (start).

Calf Raise (Calves)
(Illus. 234, 235)

This exercise also involves the simple process of rising up on your toes (lifting the heels). The resistance can be supplied by a special apparatus (a standing calf machine) or a heavy barbell across the shoulders. Again, use a block under the toes and rise up as high as possible. S-T-R-E-T-C-H. Go for 20 to 30 reps with a 50-pound barbell or use similar resistance on a special calf-machine.

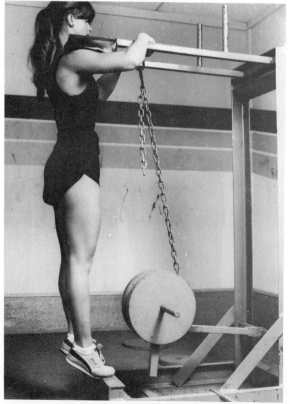

Illus. 235.   Calf raise (finish).

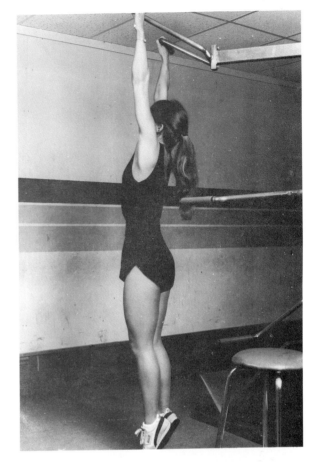

Illus. 236.   Hanging leg raise (start).

Hanging Leg Raise (**Lower Abdominals**)
(Illus. 236, 237)

This works that hard-to-get-at lower abdominal area. You'll need a horizontal bar (or a doorway chin bar) for this one. In summer a tree branch can prove adequate. Start by hanging as shown in Illus. 236. Now, with a short breath, inhale and lift the knees as shown in Illus. 237. Exhale, lower slowly, and repeat. Try 10 repetitions at first and work up over the weeks until you can perform 30.

Illus. 237.   Hanging leg raise (finish).

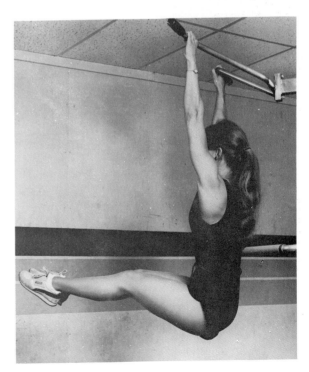

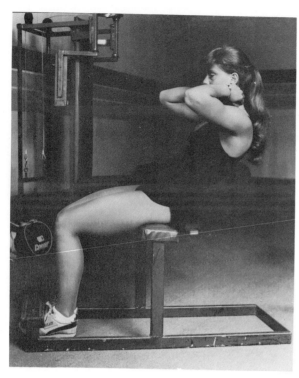

Illus. 238.   *Roman chair sit-ups (start).*

Roman Chair Sit-Ups (Abdominals)
(Illus. 238, 239)

Use a Roman chair apparatus as shown, and lower your torso slowly back. Rise up and repeat. Ten repetitions are sufficient to start. Work up until you can perform 2 or 3 sets of 25 reps.

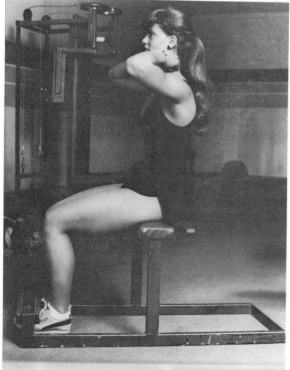

Illus. 239.   *Roman chair sit-ups (finish).*

Putting It All Together 25

It would be impossible to give you *every* exercise imaginable for each body part in this book. Although Bill Pearl's veritable treatise on weight training, *Keys to the Inner Universe*, lists thousands of exercise variations, there are still as many again to be discovered by the bodybuilders of the world.

In this book I have listed what I consider the most useful, proven exercises for each body area. Even so, you could not possibly benefit by performing *every* exercise I have listed. The job at hand now is to extract the best ones for you and "put it all together."

You cannot hope to succeed in bodybuilding without inventive thinking. You must take the knowledge imparted in these pages and use it constructively for your own bodybuilding needs. I do *not* know you. For all I know you may have huge 19-inch calves and neck while possessing a concave chest and skinny arms—or you may have a barrel chest and huge arms with virtually *no* leg development. The permutations are so limitless that it is safe to say that there is no one quite like you on the face of this earth!

Accordingly, you must learn to "see" yourself as others see you, and get busy designing a bodybuilding schedule to suit your individualized needs. I can make suggestions, but you are in charge of fine-tuning. When constructing a schedule you have to give your muscles sufficient stimulation to induce growth and at the same time avoid overtraining

which will retard your gains. You must find the balance.

Another important point: When you start a

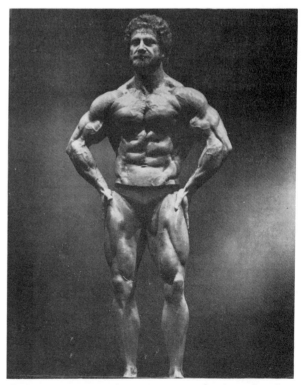

Illus. 240. Jusup Wilcosz (W. Germany) shows head-to-toe perfection.

weight-training program for the first time, always take it easy. Even if you've been training hard for years, a new exercise program can all but cripple you if you do not ease yourself into it. Start light and build up the weights and sets in each successive workout. Literally thousands of young bodybuilders have suffered excruciating aches and pains because they became overzealous during their first workout after a layoff. The body is paradoxically both strong and weak, durable and susceptible. Torn or over-worked muscles will hinder your gains. You must crawl before you can walk, and walk before you can run. Once your muscles are acclimated to your training, you can build on the experience and really let go with the heavy artillery. Indeed, you'll *have to* in order to keep your growth pattern positive.

Remember that muscle growth comes from two factors:

1. Increase in size, *not* number, of the individual muscle fibres.

2. Increase in size *and* number of the capillaries.

Muscle fibre increases in size by being subjected to a constantly heavier load. Mike Mentzer has brought this finding of medical research to the attention of the world's bodybuilders.

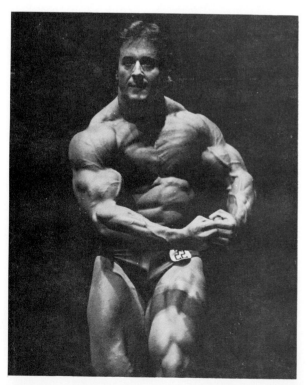

Illus. 241.   Rocky De Ferro has it all together.

Capillarization, the enlarging of the network of minute "veins" within the muscles, is brought about by utilizing plenty of sets and reps over a consistent period of regular training (average sets: 4 per exercise; 8 to 12 reps per set; 12 to 15 sets per body part.)

Most successful bodybuilders utilize both forms of training. Invariably during their *buildup* periods they will train heavily on rowing, bench press and squats and use somewhat lighter methods for other movements. Occasionally a bodybuilder will go "all-out" on every move, but this seldom leads to success because the body cannot take the stress. What would happen to you right now if you went to the gym and forced yourself to go to the limit on every exercise? You would become physically sick. If you managed to avoid actually vomiting, the chances are that the next day your system would be so over-stressed with fatigue and toxins, you would have severe diarrhea.

Some bodybuilders do have tremendous constitutions that allow them to do superhuman workouts without these unpleasant side effects. However, it should also be pointed out that often their recuperative powers are aided by taking artificial steroids, one of the few benefits of the drug. But steroids today still produce dangerous side effects of their own—sufficient reason for you to never even consider them as part of your bodybuilding program.

Here are a few programs you may want to try:

Beginners

(Start with one set only. Build up to two or three sets *after one month*)

Stretching	2 minutes
Warm-Up Rope Jumping	2 minutes
Press Behind Neck	2 × 8
Squats	2 × 8
Bench Press	3 × 8
Wide-Grip Chins	3 × 8
Barbell Curls	3 × 8
Lying Tricep Extensions	3 × 8
Standing Calf Raise	2 × 25
Crunches	2 × 12

Intermediate

Stretching	2 minutes
Warm-Up Rope Jumping	3 minutes
Press Behind Neck	3 × 8
Lateral Raise	3 × 10
Squat	4 × 10
Thigh Extension	3 × 12

Thigh Curls	3 × 15
Bench Press	3 × 8
Flyeing	4 × 10
Chin Behind Neck	3 × 12
Bent-Over Rowing	3 × 10
Barbell Curl	4 × 8
Incline Dumb-bell Curl	4 × 10
Lying Triceps Extensions	4 × 10
Triceps Pushdowns	4 × 12
Standing Calf Raise	3 × 25
Seated Calf Raise	3 × 20
Crunches	3 × 25
Hanging Leg Raise	3 × 20

Advanced

Stretching	2 minutes
Warm Up Rope Jumping	4 minutes
Press Behind Neck	4 × 8
Lateral Raise	3 × 12
Bent-Over Flyeing	3 × 12
Squat	4 × 10
Thigh Extensions	3 × 12
Thigh Curls	3 × 12
Hack Slides	3 × 12

Bench Press	4 × 8
Wide-Grip Dips	4 × 10
Flyeing	4 × 10
Chin Behind Neck	4 × 10
Barbell Rowing	4 × 10
Seated Lat Pulley Rows	3 × 12
Barbell Curl	4 × 8
Incline Dumb-bell Curl	4 × 10
Concentration Curl	4 × 12
Lying Triceps Extensions	4 × 10
Single-Arm Triceps Stretch	4 × 12
Triceps Pushdowns	4 × 12
Standing Calf Raise	4 × 25
Seated Calf Raise	4 × 25
Donkey Calf Raises	3 × 30
Crunches	3 × 25
Hanging Leg Raise	3 × 20
Prone Hyperextensions	3 × 20

Remember that these schedules are merely suggestions. Tailor your own schedule according to your own needs. Also bear in mind that if you are using *high* intensity (all-out effort), you can cut your sets to one or two per exercise: the lower your intensity, the more sets you can do.

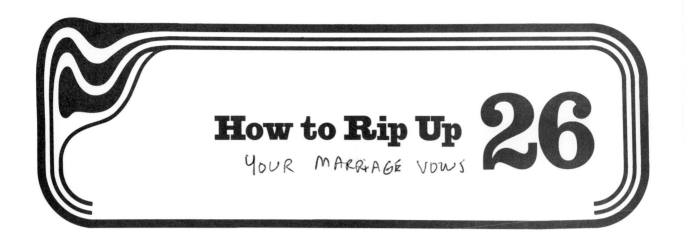

How to Rip Up 26
YOUR MARRIAGE VOWS

Probably the most important factor in winning bodybuilding contests is muscularity; formerly known as definition, today it's called "ripping up." Invariably, the most "ripped" competitor wins: seldom does the bigger man. Of course, if the biggest man is also the most ripped, then all the better for him, provided, of course, he has proportionate development.

Being ripped means one thing: possessing extremely little body fat, not just beneath the skin, but deep in the muscles themselves where fat can also accumulate, especially if your diet has been of very high caloric content. And here's the rub. Not only do you have to bring down your body fat to a very low percentage (2 to 6 percent), but you must also try to hold on to as much muscle mass as possible while reducing this body fat.

Years ago bodybuilders ripped up by keeping their protein level very high (anything from 1 to 1½ grams of protein for every pound of body weight each day.) Several top bodybuilders, including three-time Olympia winner Frank Zane and seven-time Mr. Olympia, Arnold Schwarzenegger, still use this method. But most of today's champions use less protein because excess protein will make you fat just like excess of any other food. They believe that simple calorie control will give maximum cuts, combined with hard training. You control calories by merely eating less of everything.

Frank Zane, who has to be acknowledged as the master when it comes to contest preparation, eats plenty of salads as a contest date looms. "I eat salads because of the high roughage and minerals they contain, and I use apple cider vinegar and oil as a dressing, not the commercial brands which all contain loads of sugar," he says.

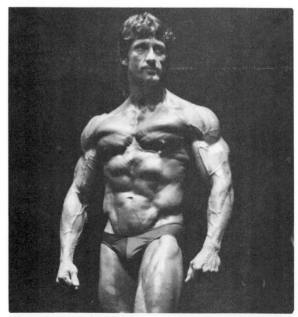

Illus. 242.   Multi-Olympia winner Frank Zane taught bodybuilders the meaning of the word ripped.

Sugar is indeed the enemy of definition. Simple sugars are found in fruit, honey, soft drinks, highly processed foods and of course table sugar. Starch and fat are a better source of energy than sugar just prior to a contest. The carbohydrates found in grains, vegetables and even potatoes contain starch and provide a much longer sustained supply of energy. Fats and starches are broken down much more slowly in the body than simple sugars. I do not mean to turn bodybuilders away from fruit during their regular training. But, because they are largely simple sugars, it may be advisable to curtail your intake of most fruit a week or two prior to the date of a contest.

Although iron man Bob Hoffman was always adamantly against bodybuilders drinking coffee, men like Steve Davis, Vince Gironda and Frank Zane, all noted for their extreme muscularity, admit to drinking it freely, especially before a contest, as the caffeine helps to curb the appetite while increasing the fat-burning process of metabolism.

It is a good idea to increase the frequency of your meals as a contest approaches. Eat every two hours, being careful to eat considerably less each time than when you ate less often. Your overall caloric intake should be gradually reduced every two weeks. Do not think that you can suddenly go from 6000 calories a day to a paltry 1000 calories. This is *not* the way to do it. Crash diets are out.

Set your goal according to the amount of fat you are carrying. A bodybuilder should never be more than 10 or 15 pounds overweight. It makes the job of getting into contest condition just too hard. If you are considerably overweight, you have to start your diet well in advance. Drop 500 calories each week. From there you will be able to gauge the degree of severity your diet must take, depending on your progress. No one can tell you how much to eat. In fact many bodybuilders peak several weeks before a contest. They then have to increase their calories slightly and try to peak at the right time by again reducing caloric intake. There certainly is no sense in peaking too early and continuing to maintain the rigid diet. You will lose too much size and on the day of the contest, your muscles will not only be too small, but they may also appear flat and unimpressive.

Other aids to muscle development such as niacin supplements (vitamin B_3), choline and inositol, liver tablets and vitamin C are mentioned in Chapter 9.

Training for definition is a very important part of your contest preparation. In days gone by, the best form of contest training was thought to be the use of a greater variety of exercises and higher repetitions. If, for example, you were using 12 exercises, 4 sets of 8 reps in your workouts, then your contest training would probably be 20 exercises, 4 sets of 15 reps. But that has all changed. The trend today is to increase intensity as the contest date approaches, much as any athlete does when a competition is approaching. High reps, especially during your precontest diet, would only cause you to lose muscular size. You would probably end up stringy and small.

If you are one of those bodybuilders who has a slow metabolism, finding that you just cannot get your fat ratio down may encourage you to cycle or run two or three days a week. Don't overdo it at first. Build up the effort until you are running 2 or 3 miles—or cycling 10 to 15 miles. Naturally, negotiating hills is a more advanced manoeuvre for both runners and cyclists. Once into it, try beating your previous time record. You will find not only that your cardiovascular health improves and you have more energy for training, especially in "long" exercises like squats, but also your endurance work will tend to speed up your metabolism of fat and you will get more muscular. Bear in mind also that as a bodybuilder you are using running for a purpose. If you run too far or too frequently, you will lose muscular size. Another substitute for running and cycling is rope-jumping. Use a good leather rope and aim to ultimately achieve a nonstop performance for 10 minutes.

It should also be added that a cutup diet of greatly limited food intake could possibly leave you short on vitamins and minerals. Therefore, I suggest in addition to any other individual vitamins you may take (such as vitamin B complex and C), you also take a daily vitamin/mineral tablet to ensure that you are getting all the essential ingredients necessary to the health of your body and its million finely-tuned functions.

Are there any exercises for cuts? The answer to this has led to a great deal of controversy in the iron game. The official medical view is that there is no such thing as spot reduction. In other words, a couple of sets of sit-ups every night isn't going to automatically give you showy "washboard" abdominals. You cannot effectively remove fat from an area by exercising it. I agree that you will burn more calories doing a set of 20 squats or go for a run than doing a few sit-ups. The more calories you burn the more fat you will get rid of over your entire body and the better the chance of having abdominals that show.

On the other hand, we have all seen long-distance runners who have extremely defined and well-muscled legs while their upper bodies have been almost devoid of muscularity because running doesn't work out the upper body. Too, we see the stringy, impressive, steel-ribbed forearms of the wheelchair athlete. The only parts void of fat are the arms, used in propelling the chair. The conclusion that even the medical profession does not refute is that spot reducing works for those who devote a great deal of effort to the task, more effort than most individuals could find time for.

And even those who could devote hours each day to spot reducing would be beaten if their overall caloric intake was so great (or the metabolism so slow) that the percentage of body fat was excessively high. One fellow I knew was training to break the world sit-up record. As a form of practice he would perform two or three *thousand* sit-ups at a time, several times weekly. But, in spite of all this he was fat. Not an ab muscle in sight. For all intents and purposes spot reducing does *not* work.

Someone in the bodybuilding game once created a stir by saying that a certain line of exercise machines "smoothed you out." An apparatus or exercise *may* smooth you out if it burns up fewer calories than you have been using with your old training methods. Let's assume you have been performing 5 sets of 20 reps in the breathing squat for a considerable time and then you get hooked on a leg machine that makes advisable only one set of substantially fewer reps, performed, unlike the squat, in the comparatively comfortable seated position. Even if the machine gives you a great feeling and you pump up like never before, you have to admit that the 5 sets of breathing squats burn up more calories. Presto! By virtue of the fact that you burn up less energy the leg machine may well smooth you out!

There is another way in which exercise can bring out your muscles—posing. There are several posing tricks you have to employ to make your presentation complete. Certain muscles have to be made prominent by posing them out because there are no totally adequate exercises to do the same job. For example: the upper thighs. The muscles that run from the upper thigh under your pose trunks do not automatically show impressiveness just because you have a low percentage of fat.

The barbell lunge exercise helps but the real

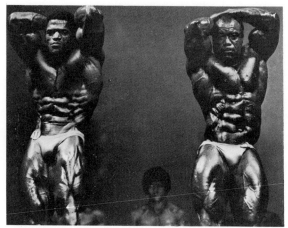

Illus. 243.   Tony Pearson and Johnny Fuller—which has the most?

credit for bringing these muscles to full glory must be given not to a formal exercise, but to those who are willing to pose the area into prominence. Spend twenty minutes a day in front of a mirror, trying to bring the area out by pushing forward, first on one foot, then the other.

Do not favor one leg more than the other. Give both limbs equal time or else you may find yourself only able to fully control the favored leg. Tom Platz, for example, the man who has the greatest leg mass and cross striations known, cannot pose his left limb as impressively as his right. The cross striations just don't show up as well. Left-legged practice will even things up in time.

You do need a low body fat percentage to allow the upper thigh muscles to show, but it is regular posing practice which really brings them out. Ask champions of upper thigh impressiveness, Steve Davis, Tony Pearson, Frank Zane and Chris Dickerson!

Other muscles which show maximum impressiveness not as a result of formal exercise, but because of posing practice are the lats (wide lats are those which have been subjected to many lat spreads, not just rowing and chinning exercises) and the *serratus* muscles (concentrate on tensing them when doing vacuums, lat spreads and double biceps poses).

Also, pecs which have a good "roll" (the flexed rippling muscles of thick, well-developed pecs) and "split" (the separation between tensed upper and lower pecs) are usually that way as a result of posing and "crunching" (eliminating air from lungs while sucking in waist) rather than the usual run of chest exercises.

How to Prepare for a Contest 27
BAND

Preparing for a contest must, of course, be predicated upon your having acquired at least a fair build. You cannot enter a bodybuilding contest if you just don't have any development. It is also useless to even contemplate entering a competition unless the muscles you do have show up as *muscles* and not fat-covered bulk! After which all glory comes from daring to begin. You must decide ahead of time which contest you are going to enter. It's no good entering the Mr. America contest if you haven't even won your area contest. Your first contest should be a novice show. The longer you have to prepare, the better your chances. Be content to make haste slowly.

You should first find out what contests are all about. If you haven't even seen one, do so. Attend both the evening show and the prejudging. Most bodybuilding contests are judged earlier in the day because it is difficult for judges to come up with a fair conclusion in the rush of the evening's procedures. Perhaps the top few men are relatively easy to pick out, but ranking the other contestants in order of merit is more difficult and time-consuming. The more leisurely prejudging period allows judges more time to scrutinize and compare physiques and the relative strengths and weaknesses of the contestants.

By attending a couple of shows, you will find out what is expected of you. You will not only get a pretty good idea of how strong the competition is,

but also better understand what cannot be overemphasized—that the act of posing *makes or breaks* a bodybuilding competitor. Do it poorly and you will fail; do it superbly and the winner's trophy could be yours.

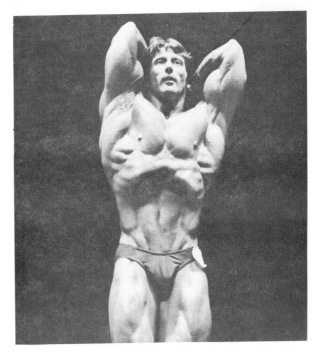

Illus. 244.   Frank Zane, multi-Olympia winner is always tanned to maximum when he enters competition.

Depending on how much lead time you have, divide your plan of action into phases. The exact plan will depend on a large variety of factors. As an example, if you are really overweight, you had better start a strict diet right away. If you are on the thin side with no fat problem, you can keep your calories pretty high until close to the event.

Frank Zane has a three-phase plan for entering shows:

Phase One

Here, Zane uses very heavy poundages and works each body part twice a week.

Phase Two

The transition period, which is geared to moving from size training to separation training by adding one workout a week.

Phase Three

Frank puts the finishing touches on his physique by bringing out the cuts within the muscle itself and trying to use the same poundages while reducing caloric intake.

Only you can judge how long each phase must last. There is no universal blueprint for success. It might be a good idea to set a target date for a photo session sometime during the summer. Plan your preparation carefully and see if you can peak on a certain day. It is not an easy thing to do. Many bodybuilders have found that they have either peaked too early or else they just couldn't make it at all. There are thousands of bodybuilders every year, even some professionals, who go through the arduous process of preparing for a contest only to not turn up on the day of the show. Reason? They couldn't manage to peak for the event!

But once a bodybuilder learns how to do it, he will never forget. In a nutshell, one has to progressively increase workout intensity *and* training frequency while decreasing caloric intake sufficiently to eat up the fat content of the body and at the same time maintain maximum muscle mass.

It is important to sunbathe the body as the contest date approaches. Do this over a period of the last month. Do not make the mistake of thinking that you can tan up in a day or two prior to the event. This is impossible. The body needs to darken progressively over a period to a deep nut-brown hue. A friend of mine, John Mikl (a Mr. Canada winner), flew down to Las Vegas prior to entering a big con-

test. He lay in the desert sun for two days and then returned to enter the show. He didn't manage it. His body was so burnt and swollen he entered a hospital instead. His lesson was well learned. Today John tans up for several weeks before the contest. Even black bodybuilders like Chris Dickerson, Serge Nubret and Rick Wayne have to sunbathe prior to a show. All three have pale olive-colored skin, but after a week or two in the sun, they look like bronzed gods.

It is important to sunbathe *all* parts of the body, particularly under the arms and the sides of the legs, two of the most neglected areas. Accordingly, spend a good percentage of your sunbathing time lying with your underarms exposed to the rays. But be *sure* to apply *sunscreen all over* to filter out harmful rays that cause burning and are implicated in skin cancer and early wrinkling. You will still tan well but *gradually*. Do not do a great deal of sunning in the seated position. The creases will show across your abdomen.

Those of you who just cannot get a good tan may have to resort to coloring lotion. It is still wise to sunbathe and get some type of coloring even if only on the pink side, because most bottled tans look less than perfect when spread over lily-white skin that has barely seen the light of day from one year to the next.

Another word of warning: Apply any artificial bottled tan in "layers" with a facecloth. Put on one layer and allow to dry, then add another, and another, and so on. You have to experiment with this well before the show. It cannot be left to chance, nor can you rely on it looking right if you haven't experimented beforehand. Two noticeably bad mistakes were apparent at a local contest I judged recently. One guy had made a bad choice of bottle tan. He appeared on stage as positively "orange." We needed sunglasses just to look at him. Another fellow hadn't considered the effect oil would have when rubbed over his artificial color. The streaking effect made him look more like a zebra than a human being. In his case it was a pity because he had the muscles to pull off a convincing win. But he didn't.

Posing in front of an audience can be unnerving. Certainly it is hard to feel at ease, let alone actually enjoy the experience. The trick of course is not to enjoy it but to *appear* to enjoy it.

Practice, practice and practice some more. Get a trusted and knowledgeable friend to appraise your routine. If he tells you it is perfect, drop him. He's not telling you the truth. Find someone who cares about you and will offer constructive criticism. Remember that the system you are judged by may require you to perform certain compulsory poses, like standard lat spreads, double biceps, side chests, abdominal, back and thigh poses.

In your free posing, the poses of your own choice you perform, it is important that each attitude not only show your body to advantage, but hide any weakness you may have. For example, if you feel that you do not have enough size, don't stretch out your legs and arms like a ballet dancer. You should adopt more compact poses that do not draw attention to your undersized limbs. Try for the most part to keep your arms close to your body, and never spread your legs out too far. Some bodybuilders who have weak or under-par legs adopt numerous poses that only show the legs from the side, or else they perform crouched or kneeling poses to hide their flawed legs.

Many bodybuilders do not have a very impressive biceps peak. So what should they do? The question, of course, should be: What should they *not* do? They should not make it obvious that they lack biceps peak by constantly flexing up their biceps!

Of course, this artful posing can and should work both ways. If you find that you have an exceptional body part, by all means exploit it. Former Mr. Olympia Larry Scott had superb arms and made the most of them in almost every pose he adopted. Other super bodybuilders such as Frank Zane and Chris Dickerson could be described as slightly lacking in arm size. Both men, nevertheless, have won scores of the world's top titles. Each man has developed a posing routine of such phenomenal individuality and finesse that any weaknesses are totally obliterated by comparison.

One important aspect of posing is muscle growth. Just bending your arms and flexing is not enough. You must develop complete all-around muscle control. This means that you must practice posing until you can flex your thighs as well as your arms, your abdominal muscles, back, *serratus*, calves—all while faking a smile that tells the audience (and judges) that you're enjoying every minute, when in fact you are tensing and concentrating like hell to bring about the desired effect.

Another aspect of posing is to make your presentation in an exciting manner. You need to know what you are doing and put the whole thing over with verve and originality. The sport of bodybuilding is full of young hopefuls who hover from one pose to another while on stage. Often each pose is followed by a lengthy pause where the contestant shuffles his feet and is obviously lost as to what the next pose is going to be. This is no way to make a powerful impression. There is no way to change from pose to pose. You can glide into it, slide into it, rip into it, zip into it—but whatever you do, you must make it appear planned and deliberate. The posing platform is no place for indecision or amateurism. You must come across like a polished pro.

Even the color of your pose briefs is important. Never wear any type of patterned or striped trunks. You are trying to sell the judges on your body, not your pose briefs. Stay with plain colors, usually the richer tones rather than the lighter shades such as powder blue, yellow or peach. The most popular colors at present are maroon and tan, but many contestants find that certain colors like sea blue complement their skin coloring and make for a pleasing overall effect. Dark blues are popular as are black trunks, although I must admit an aversion to black trunks which I feel seldom add sufficient emphasis to a physique. Black is such a nondescript tone, totally lacking in forcefulness of statement.

For the most part, your pose trunks should be "high cut" at the thigh because you need to display the upper thigh muscles to win a big show. Low-cut (straight-across) trunks do not show the upper thigh muscles well and also serve to "kill the line" of the overall leg appearance.

Remember to look confident while you pose, in fact all the time you are on stage. Try not to look down at your torso. You may have to check once or twice to see that the light is falling across your pecs and abdominals in the right manner, but there is a heck of a difference between a competitor who allows himself a couple of quick, one-second glances

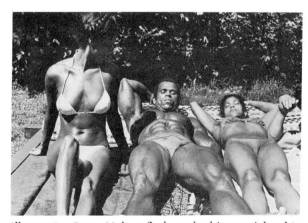

Illus. 245.   Serge Nubret finds sunbathing enriches his skin color and tone to help set off his physique.

145

and one who spends half his time with head bowed looking at himself. Such insecurity! Is he worried that his muscles are going to deflate and disappear from sight right there on stage?

Although you will not always be allowed to pose to your own choice of music, it is nevertheless a good idea to practice posing to some of your favorite pieces. Choose the most inspiring music you can find. You need to pose to the kind of music that "moves the crowd." They must feel part of your act, inspired, not only by your unique posing ability, but by the fantastic musical accompaniment you are using to project your routine and your superior body development.

The bodybuilder's diet prior to a contest is vitally important. He doesn't have to be an expert in nutrition, but he does have to be expertly disciplined. For most bodybuilders the precontest diet is the hardest and most gruelling part of the training. As the weeks dwindle away towards contest time, so must your food intake. Ultimately, most competitive bodybuilders will go from eating virtually anything their hearts desire for months prior to show date to eating only egg whites, fish (boiled), turkey and water during the last few weeks. Here is a three-stage diet that is typical for today's hardcore bodybuilder.

Four Months Prior to Contest Date

BREAKFAST	MORNING SNACK	LUNCH	AFTERNOON SNACK	SUPPER	EVENING SNACK
cereal	cheese	glass of	mixed fruit	steak	soup
bacon	sandwich	milk	coffee	potatoes	cheese or
sausage		steak and		vegetables	meat
eggs		egg sandwich		dessert	sandwich
toast		fruit		coffee	
honey		ice cream			
coffee					

Two Months Prior to Contest Date
(No sugar, salt)

BREAKFAST	MORNING SNACK	LUNCH	AFTERNOON SNACK	SUPPER	EVENING SNACK
six-egg	one piece	cold beef	coffee	steak	two-egg
omelette	of fruit	cuts		tomatoes	omelette
1 slice	(apple,	fresh fruit		spinach	
of toast	banana, etc.)				
coffee					

Two Weeks Prior to Contest Date
(No sugar, coffee cream, salt)

BREAKFAST	MORNING SNACK	LUNCH	AFTERNOON SNACK	SUPPER	EVENING SNACK
6 to 10	water	can of water-	water	turkey or	water
boiled or		packed tuna		chicken,	
poached		or boiled		broiled	
eggs		whitefish		(not fried)	
vitamin-mineral		plain green		plain green	
supplements		salad (no		salad (no	
coffee		dressing)		dressing	

146

One last point: It is essential to shave off all excess body hair prior to entering a bodybuilding contest, in order to get your muscles to show up to advantage. This is best done with soap and water and plenty of razors. Do not leave it until the last day. It is far better to shave the body and legs a couple of times during the week of the show rather than leave the entire job until the last hours. You could get razor burns or an allergic reaction which would show up when you least wanted attention drawn to the problem. Do not use chemical or cream preparations to rid yourself of body hair. They can spoil skin appearance.

The Art and Drama of Posing 28

Posing is the essence of bodybuilding: As Charles Gaines wrote in his excellent book, *Pumping Iron*, "Posing is the heart of this thing. Depending on how it is done, you can see in it either everything that is moving and beautiful and dignified about the display of a developed body or everything that is ridiculous and embarrassing about it."

The prime reason for posing is to show what you've got. There are side benefits too, not the least of which are added muscular size, shape and definition. Posing brings out the "cuts." Although posing packs its greatest punch when the physique is truly balanced and conditioned, it is not unusual for a skilled bodybuilder to hide otherwise glaring faults with a good posing routine set off by dynamic and inspiring music.

Since the nineteenth century when Sandow would dust white powder on his muscles before entering a special posing booth (he was proud of his white skin but believed in being whiter than white) and then, more often than not, "for ladies only," would pose during his music hall act around the world, posing has been increasingly important in the world of physical culture.

After Sandow came Sig Klein and Tony Sanson, both of New York City and John Carl Grimek of York, Pennsylvania, the "Monarch of Muscledom." Grimek did not have quite the sharpness of today's bodybuilders, but he could really pose and he had the size and the tan. (Somehow the vogue has changed from being as white as possible to being as dark as possible. As mentioned before, even black bodybuilders sunbathe prior to a contest to give the skin a rich color and healthy texture.) Grimek's routine (mainly during the '40s and '50s) was recognized as a complete work of art. Rumor has it that Grimek had a girlfriend who was an accomplished ballerina and learned much about the art of physical display from her. Whether or not this is true, Grimek was a mas-

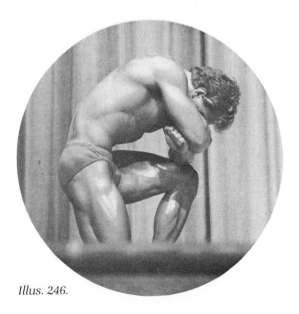

Illus. 246.

148

ter. Bob Hoffman's *Strength and Health* magazine was an inspiration to the world's bodybuilders during the twenty years following World War II. Thousands would simply not buy the magazine unless a new picture of the immortal "Jawn" appeared in its pages.

One incident which lent authority to Grimek's reputation as the world's greatest poser (and proves his versatility) happened at the Mr. Universe contest in London, England way back in 1948. Grimek versus Reeves; you couldn't have picked two more different physical types. Grimek, relatively short (5'9"), compact, sporting huge melon-sized shoulders, full "riding-britches" thighs, a thick barrel chest and enormous 19-inch arms contrasted sharply to the equally-bronzed Reeves, standing over 6 feet tall with wide, "rangy" shoulders. Lacking Grimek's eye-popping density throughout his entire physique, Reeves somehow made amends with his superb line, handsomeness and unquestionably proportionate body.

After each had posed once before the audience, the judges were in a quandary. They were equally divided between the two men. To break the deadlock it was decreed that both Reeves and Grimek should pose once more. First Reeves, with his masculine beauty and almost unreal proportions, repeated his repertoire to the delirious applause of the London crowd, and then—John Carl Grimek. What followed made bodybuilding history. John gave the audience and judges something totally different. Instead of repeating his routine as Reeves had done, he performed an entirely different selection of mind-blowing poses, ultimately back-flipping off the rostrum and tossing himself to the ground in a full split. Pandemonium reigned. Applause and cheers battered against the walls and roof of the theatre and poured in wave after wave towards the now victorious Grimek. It was one of those moments in bodybuilding that will not be forgotten.

As the '40s gave way to the '50s we saw a new more formal era, championed by Britisher Reg Park. To the perennial strains of "The Legend of the Glass Mountain" Reg would perform first an arty "stretched-out" stance and then a "brutal" basic muscle pose, believing that by their contrast, each would lend weight and drama to the other. Because of this, and what was considered the greatest physique on earth, Reg was greatly in demand throughout the world as a guest posing attraction. His fee, outrageous at the time, was fifty pounds—two hundred dollars. It was, of course, gladly paid because Reg Park on the bill virtually guaranteed a full house

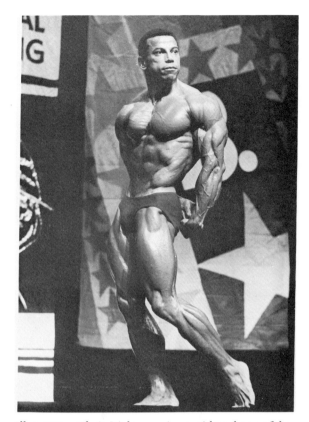

Illus. 247.   Chris Dickerson is considered one of the all-time great posers.

at show time. Today, top pro bodybuilders demand from between $1,000 to $5,000 (plus travel expenses) for a five-minute guest spot. Currently our most inspiring posers are Chris Dickerson, Frank Zane and Ed Corney, each now on the verge of retirement since both Zane and Dickerson are over forty and Corney has topped the half-century mark. Who will follow?

There is a curious thing about posing: It is very hard for a bodybuilder to pose effectively unless he feels "right" about his physical condition that day. A great poser can definitely "go off." I can remember seeing Reg Park in 1956 guest posing at the N.A.B.B.A. Mr. Universe contest at the London Palladium. His act was an awe-inspiring work of art. A few years later, posing to the same music, Park's posing was sloppy and disjointed. He even readjusted his trunks a couple of times during the routine, all because he did not feel at his best. Several years later Reg Park was back on target again.

The same thing happened to Hawaiian Ed Corney. He emerged as a physique star around 1974, because of his sensational posing. Almost overnight

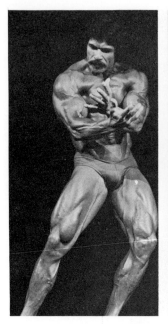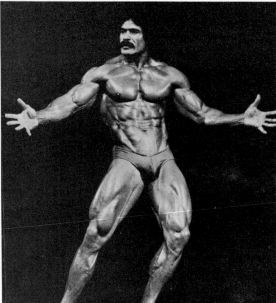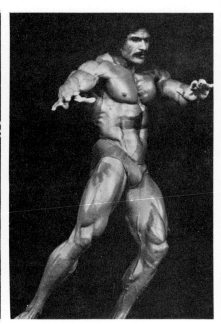

Illus. 248–252.   A sequence of poses by the grand master—Hawaii's Ed Corney.

he was acclaimed "the world's greatest poser." Corney's glide from one position to another was sheer magic. He never quite possessed an Olympia-winning physique, but on more than one occasion he *almost* took the title from the big boys. Wherever he went, Corney got the loudest ovations and invariably was the crowd's favorite because of his stupendous posing routine. He would "feel" his way from one pose to another, often grabbing at the air and twisting from one position to another. He could go from a back pose to a front pose and you would hardly see his feet move. Although he was always immensely popular, for some reason Corney changed his routine. Erroneously, he concluded that the public perhaps wanted a change. Nothing could be further from the truth. Since the day he decided to change his routine, Ed Corney has not managed to set the crowds afire as he used to.

The standard way of posing is to walk on stage, climb one or two steps to a dais or posing plinth, position yourself under the spotlight and adopt about ten to fifteen poses that show your physique off to advantage, concluding inevitably with the most muscular or "crab" position. That is the standard way. It is not the *best* way. To win contests today, you have to have a dynamic pose routine that incorporates everything. That is to say you must show muscle size, proportion, facial confidence, zest

and ambition, a complete head-to-toe tan, muscular separation, definition, appealing shape and line, and of course artistry and drama in bringing off each and every pose as an aesthetic masterpiece in its own right.

After your panic subsides, let's analyze each factor:

Muscle Size

Adequate muscle size is pretty important because the sport is *bodybuilding* and it's no good entering a contest unless you are *built!* On the other hand, you do not have to have 22-inch upper arms to win. Many prize-winning bodybuilders have won the most prestigious contests in the world with arms barely exceeding 17½ inches. Frank Zane and Chris Dickerson are two such examples.

A bodybuilder in shape is not a huge man. Often he looks almost "small" in clothes. Frequently at physique contests I see people in the audience who look to be just about twice as big as anyone on stage competing, but there's a difference. The giants in clothes would look ordinary on stage because the bodybuilders are cut to ribbons, but in all probability the Goliaths are carrying thirty pounds of blubber—or more! Basic size, not hugeness, is necessary.

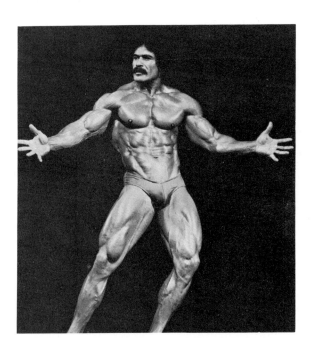
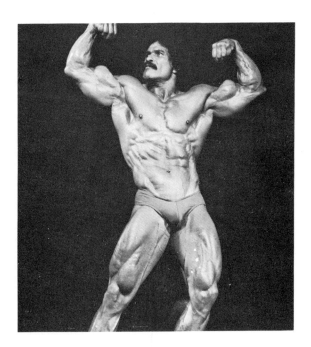

Proportion

Entering a contest with poor body proportion, or lack of symmetry if you like, is asking for trouble. Often you will see bodybuilders at physique meets with very slight calf development or perhaps a "narrow" back which doesn't flair out in typical bodybuilder fashion. You will look less than spectacular if you are not proportionately built. Underdeveloped thighs or poorly developed chests often solicit such remarks from other bodybuilders such as "He's got no legs" or "He has no chest at all," this in spite of the fact that you may have 26-inch thighs and a 50-inch chest. If these body parts are not impressive, cut, split and muscular, in the eyes of your bodybuilding colleagues they don't even exist. I will always remember Frank Zane telling me his opinion of Arnold when Schwarzenegger first came to America. The two had just met in the Miami IFBB Mr. Universe in which the more "finished" Zane had beaten the Austrian. Arnold had big shoulders and pecs and enormous arms, but insignificant ab development and somewhat under par legs. There was some controversy about the decision since Zane was not noted for size (which Arnold did possess for the most part) and yet the Oak's definition could have been better while Zane's was famous. The remark that Zane made to justify the decision? "Arnold has absolutely nothing below the pecs—nothing!"

Facial Confidence

The successful bodybuilder must exude confidence on stage. It has to be obvious from his walk, his demeanor and above all, his face. This does not mean that you have to scoff at your fellow competitors or show your teeth in every pose. But confidence, even if it is not there in your heart, must *seem* to be there for the judges. So often I see contestants with their heads hanging low nervously twitching as though they have ants in their pants, eyeballing their pecs and abs with seeming fear that they might vanish before their eyes.

Apart from a cursory glance to check that the light is right, never look at yourself when on stage. You should have your head held high facing the judges or out to the audience, but never be caught checking out your pecs—keep that for the gym or the bathroom mirror.

Zest and Ambition

One of the golden rules of salesmanship is to *ask for the order*. If you're selling something to a potential buyer, don't just mumble about the product's merits. Come out straight and ask for the order: "I would like you to buy this product from me." Say it! Ask!

On stage in competition you are the salesman.

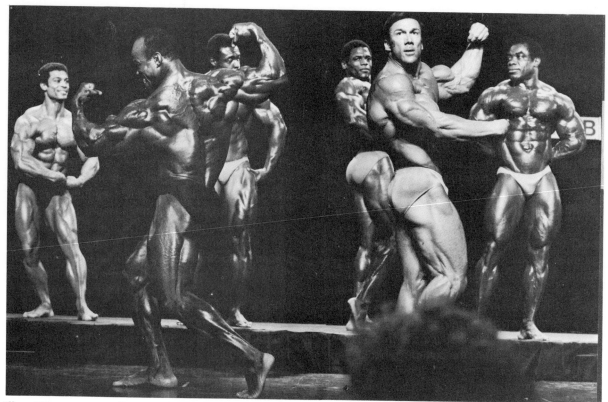

Illus. 253.   *At pose-off time everyone does their things.*

You cannot play the part of an "also ran!" You have to show everybody who matters that you are serious about winning the contest. This is probably the one time in your life where you *have* to get physically aggressive.

Assert yourself. Be prepared to do battle with each and every competitor who is a challenge. Dominate the stage. During the posedowns you should be the first to pose and the last to stop posing. Champions of *aggressive* posing, really nice guys to know *off* the bodybuilding stage, are Ron Teufel and Tom Platz. The all-time "fighter" is Tony Pearson. He never gives in. Even against men like Oliva, Johns and Fox, Pearson will wrench every drop of sweat from his body by just refusing to quit posing until his opponents all but collapse in their own pools of sweat.

Tanning

Whether it comes from a bottle or from the sun, color is very important to the modern bodybuilder at contest time. You must be a deep bronze from head to toe and under the arms. See the previous chapter for a fuller discussion of tanning methods.

Muscular Separation

This phenomenon is more important today than ever. Separation is the clarity of division between the various muscles that make up the external physique. In the '50s, a thigh, for example, was considered pretty good if it had a couple of slices and a lump or two in its upper reaches. Today a thigh is great only if it has perfectly defined quads, *vastus internus*, *vastus externus*, totally delineated abductor muscles, fully curved thigh biceps and, of course, cross-striated muscles from top to bottom.

Separation means that your delts must jump out from your shoulders, and cut sharply into the upper arms. Separation means sharply outlined *serratus* and intercostals. Separation means abdominals that show below the belly button, oblique ridges that tuck under the trunks at the top, and upper thigh muscles that pop out of the trunks at the bottom. Separation is head-to-toe muscles that could be mistaken for a den of serpents.

Definition

Fat under the skin is the arch enemy of muscular definition. The lower the percentage of body fat, the greater will be the show of muscle. Also, although not all bodybuilders desire it in excess, your vascularity too will be more prominent. It goes without saying that if you have paper-thin skin (little or no fat), your muscles will show up to a great degree. The phenomenon of "cross striations" are a result of greatly improved definition. Of course you have to bear in mind that even the thinnest skin cannot reveal muscles or cross striations if they are not there in the first place.

Vascularity is part and parcel of definition; the veins show up clearly, but like cross striations, they are more visible in the physiques of those bodybuilders who call upon the aid of artificial steroid drugs to build their body. Steroids which are dealt with in Chapter 10 are not recommended.

Shape and Line

You are not going to impress anyone without possessing a good shape and attractive line. Shape, to a great extent, is inherited, dependent on your natural allotment of cells and on bone size and never shows up to advantage unless you have a minimum of body fat.

Line is both inherited and acquired. You may have good natural line, but continuous, unbalanced training could take it away. If, on the other hand, throughout your career you pay particular attention to your weak points, working them harder (and longer) than your easier growing areas, you will maximize your chances of making your overall line as good as it can possibly be.

Artistry and Drama

Posing is *made* by these two elements. You need to interest the audience and the judges. Whether you do this with slow, deliberate posing, dynamic, fast, sweeping motions, or whether you choose to change the pace of your routine midway and adopt classical, brutal, ballet-like, Herculean, charismatic or awesome poses, you call the shots. The free-posing section of a bodybuilding contest is your chance to impress, to show what you can do. Posing at its worst will see a bodybuilder shuffling his feet, straining to remember what to do next, contorting his face in pain, huffing, puffing and shaking from the effort, and ultimately adopting uninspiring, bad and boring attitudes.

At its *best* posing can bring an audience to its feet and even bring unbridled cheers from the show officials, photographers and judges alike. Get it right and you can hold the crowd in the palm of your hand

as you slide from pose to pose, creating never-to-be-forgotten frames of dynamic muscularity.

Since you usually pose to music, sometimes you may be lucky enough, or famous enough, to pose to your own choice of music, a record or tape you have often used in practice. Your choice of music should be made with care, for maximum impact on your particular routine. Chris Dickerson, the currently acknowledged "World's Greatest Poser" has used numerous vocal recordings, but his most successful to my mind was Dionne Warwick's "I Know I'll Never Love This Way Again." Other favorites that have the right touch of tear-jerking inspirational melodrama are "Born Free," "Rocky," "Exodus" and "Superman" although these four latter themes have been somewhat overused by the bodybuilding professionals of the day. Champions like Boyer Coe and Frank Zane often use hard rock music like "Pink Floyd," which has an advantage over other themes in that its loudness is not easily superseded by the audience's vociferous, foot-stomping approval.

One of the best musically orchestrated demonstrations I have ever seen was made by Samir Bannout. The name of the theme escapes me, but it commences in a soft manner, with birds singing and chirping, at which time you could be forgiven for

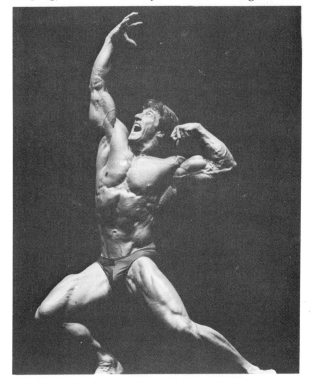

Illus. 254.   Dynamic is the word for Frank Zane, three-time Mr. Olympia.

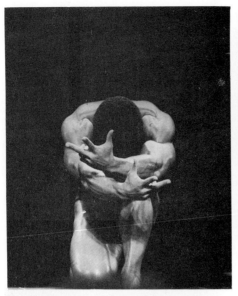
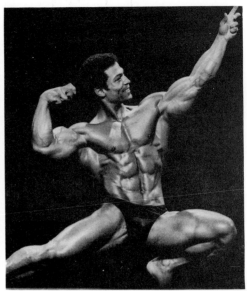
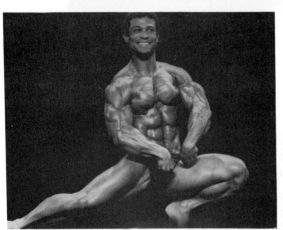
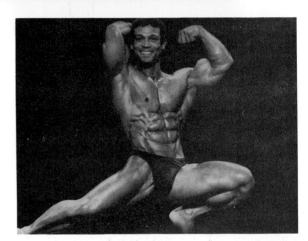
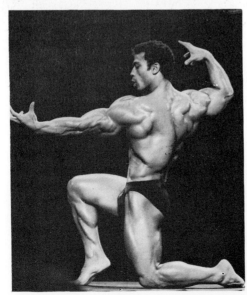

Illus. 255–264.   Egypt's Mohamed Makkawy brings the aesthetic posing of another continent to American bodybuilding in this sequence.

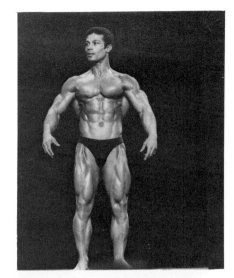
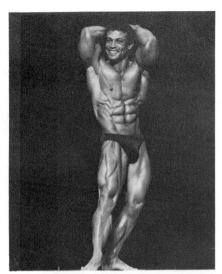
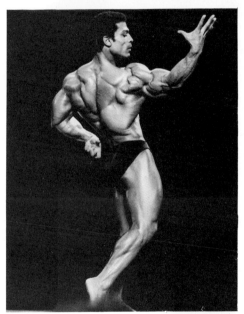
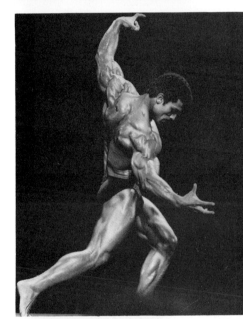

JANINE'S
CONDUCTING
PROF

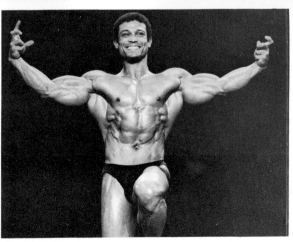

stifling a yawn. During this introduction Bannout raises his arms and "fixes in" on several aesthetic attitudes for which he is famous, and then it happens. The chirping ceases and the rhythm of the music flings itself into high gear with a series of tumultuous chimes, each of which sees Samir in a new dynamic muscular pose. Tears appear in the eyes of the audience; screams accompany each new attitude. The demonstration is sensational, and leaves the incredulous crowd with all but bleeding hands and a hoarseness that will last a week!

Posing done properly should mask flaws in your physique. Arnold Schwarzenegger, known for being the world's best built man during the '70s, would be the first to admit that his physique has inherent faults which he can only hope to disguise rather than eliminate entirely. His waist and hips are boxy, his upper thighs are never really cut up, the calves are knotty and certainly not aesthetically shaped, one thigh biceps has a lump which not even *Gray's Anatomy* has on record and his triceps are just not in line with his enormous biceps development. Yet Arnold is still the world's number one favorite because he still has more pluses and fewer minuses than all the others.

Serge Nubret and Dennis Tinerino share more than the fact that they are often referred to as the uncrowned Mr. Olympias. Both have very impressive

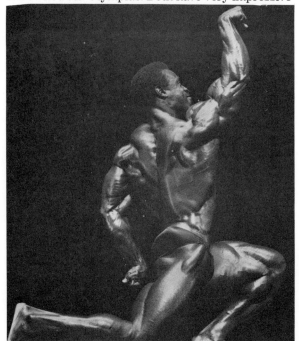

Illus. 265.   Roy Callender (Canada) in his most famous pose.

physiques in the relaxed (standing hands by the side) position. But weaknesses begin to appear when they pose. Both lose the massiveness from their arms when raised in the traditional double-biceps pose, so you will find that only when called upon to show their arms will they adopt this position. The most flattering poses for both men are those in which the arms are held close to the body. Likewise with their backs. Both Nubret and Tinerino have phenomenal backs in the relaxed position, but the arms-above-head pose takes away the important massiveness. Men like Arnold or Franco of course could pose their arms without *losing* their backs because they had untold density to spare.

The calf is a particularly hard area to hide as it is seen from almost any angle. It is important to work the hell out of them, at least as hard as you work your arms, to progressively build up the poundage resistance week by week. There is also something else you can do, a trick that both Tony Pearson and Robby Robinson adopted. They *lessened* the size of their upper legs, with the result that the smaller thigh with its shallower sweep flowed better into the calf area and the size discrepancy was less noticeable.

The only way to improve your posing is to pose often. Take off time after a workout to repeat your routine several times, and always try new poses. Of particular importance are basic poses such as the double biceps, the lat spread (from front and back) and the side chest and side triceps poses.

A pose may not suit you at first, but constant practice will *make* it right. At one time Frank Zane dreaded the lat spread. He just didn't look right doing it and lost contests perhaps because it wasn't one of his better poses. In the mid-'70s, however, he decided he would master the lat spread, and practiced it ceaselessly. The result: It is now one of his *super* poses, which he does as well as anyone else in bodybuilding.

Regular posing will not only make your lats "come out," it will sharpen your *serratus*, intercostals and abs and add a splendor to your thighs you may have not thought possible. Most bodybuilders known for their upper thigh detail brought it out by determined regular posing of that area.

That's true of the pecs also. Franco Columbu, who has contracted his pecs more than anyone, has the biggest and most noticeable pectoral split. In today's contests, posing ability is more than just the icing on the cake—it plays a very important part in building, shaping and dramatizing your body.

The Day of the Show 29

Always turn up on time at a show. Nothing is worse than having to rush to get into your trunks because you are late arriving. It is a good idea to check the exact location of the pre-judging hall or theatre some days before the contest so you will be able to know exactly what you are doing on the day you need to know.

It is customary for bodybuilders to virtually starve right up until contest time and then to load up on carbohydrates the morning of the contest. When I say *load up*, I do not mean that they have five plates of spaghetti (that comes after the contest). Carbohydrate loading means that a bodybuilder will consume a single baked potato or a carbohydrate "goodie" of similar size. This prevents the muscles from looking too flat on the day of the show. It may also help to eliminate excessive shaking when posing and definitely contributes towards helping you obtain a good pump prior to letting the judges see your physique.

What is pumping? It is the performance of low intensity exercises using very little resistance for high repetitions (20 to 40 reps). Usually it is best to pump using movements that you do not normally perform in your regular workouts. And do them as fast as possible. Typical pumping moves are floor dips, parallel bar dips, chins, and strand exercises.

And what about the pump? Is it necessary to pump up the muscles before going on stage? One man who always got a great pump, in fact just about

performed a full workout, was Sergio Oliva. On occasion he would spend over an hour flushing his muscles before a contest. At one show he was competing in, the N.A.B.B.A. Mr. Universe, much to the amazement of spectators and judges alike, Oliva visibly shrank while standing on stage. He had obtained his usual enormous pump, but while standing on stage waiting for the other competitors to go through their individual routines, the size gradually left him.

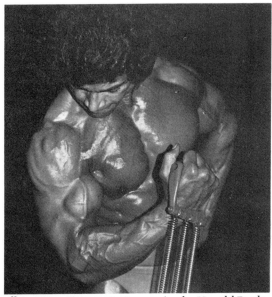

Illus. 266.   Pre-contest pumping by Harold Poole.

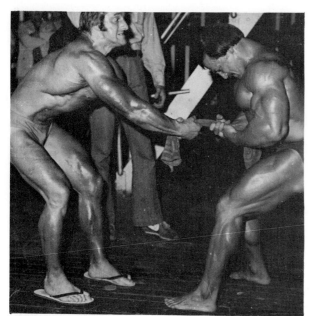

Illus. 267.   Holding a towel. The backstage pumping ritual begins.

Bill Pearl seldom pumped up before entering a contest. He would just go through his posing routine a couple of times and generally relax until called on stage. His philosophy: "If I don't have it now, I never will!"

The act of pumping before a show can be good and bad. Certainly excessive pumping can lessen your chances of victory. Because it is gorged with blood, a highly pumped muscle *loses* definition. Also you can lose your ability to flex or control your muscles if they are over-pumped. Certainly you can make your arms bigger by pumping them up, but you will also round out your biceps and lose biceps height (peak) if you overdo it. Likewise the triceps can lose impressive delineation if excessively pumped. They will appear, and be, bulkier, but detail, especially when the arm is straightened, will not be so evident.

Traditionally, bodybuilders would really go to town pumping their pectoral muscles prior to going on stage. This is not done so much today because the pecs are seldom a region that is lacking in size, as used to be the case years ago before the advent of sophisticated adjustable bench apparatus, Pek-Deks, chest machines and the like. Nor is it suggested that "lowers" such as forearms and calves be pumped because these areas seldom pump up to a noticeable increase in size. Besides, these two areas, if heavily pumped, could cramp up during your posing display. The best areas to pump are:

THE LATS

With a towel and a partner you can indulge in some bent-over pulling to work the lats. Alternatively, many competitors chin or even row. Fully-pumped lats are an advantage in a contest.

THE TRICEPS

Pump them fairly well, but do not *overgorge* them with blood. Best exercises: close-grip pushups, parallel bar dips, or back press with strands.

PECS

These will usually pump up along with the triceps and lat exercises, and unless your pecs are definitely lacking in size, you should not pump them up fully.

THIGHS AND CALF

You could do a few squats to get the blood flowing in your legs, but generally speaking, if you don't have the size by now, there's not much you can do that will change things . . . except to resolve to squat harder during the coming year.

DELTOIDS

Definitely worth pumping hard here. The shoulders do not suffer too much loss of definition when pumped and do add impressiveness and width to the physique. Pump them fully with short nonlock barbell presses, upright rows, and laterals with weights or strands.

TRAPS

Pump only if this is a weak area. Best exercise: shrugs.

Unless the rules state that you must not wear oil, you had better make sure yours is applied profes-

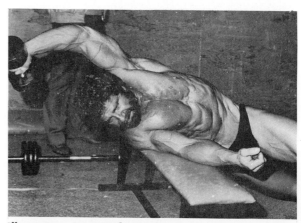

Illus. 268.   Jusup Wilcosz showing a unique pumping exercise he performs before going on stage.

sionally, that is to say, evenly. You need someone else to apply oil on your back. It should be lightly rubbed in, not poured on and ·spread around like butter. A heavy coating of oil will reflect too many highlights and can actually make you appear smooth if you are slightly smooth already. If you are really in shape and ripped, a huge load of oil will not smooth you out, but neither will it help your general appearance because you will look just like a walking mirror, blinding the audience and judges with reflected light.

At the show's conclusion when the winners are announced, if you don't place as high as you think you should, don't make a scene. It's a good lesson in sportsmanship. Grit your teeth and bear it. Resolve to train harder during the coming year so that next time there will be no doubt that you should be the overall winner. There are some contests that for one reason or another do not come up with the best decisions. History has crowned some atrocious winners. And yes, some contests *are* fixed and others for one reason or another *appear* to be fixed when in fact they are not.

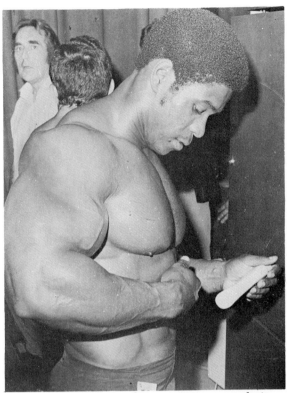

Illus. 270.   Britain's Bertil Fox uses a cream solution to soften highlights.

Illus. 271.   The incredible Mike Mentzer gets help in oiling himself prior to competing in the Olympia event

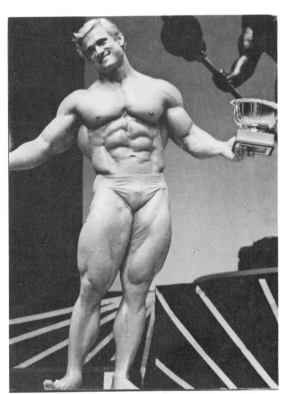

Illus. 269.   No one takes a second place win better than Platz, even when the audience tells him he should have won.

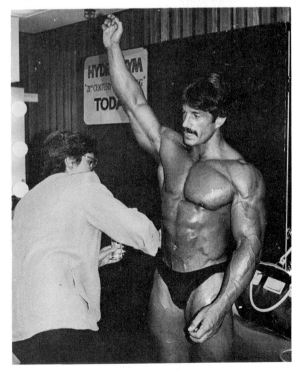

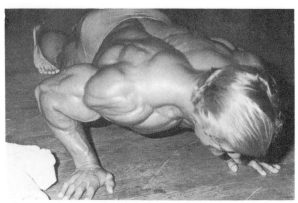

Illus. 272.   Tom Platz resorts to the basic pushup prior to being judged on stage.

But fortunately for the amateur, there is a greater chance of the best man winning. This extends to the AAU Mr. America title held continuously since 1939, a prestigious contest where for the most part, and with only few exceptions, the best man of the day was awarded the title.

It is regrettable that as a competing bodybuilder, you will often be told by your "friends" that you had "the best physique in the show!" or, if you failed to win, "You were robbed!" In the thirty years I have spent around bodybuilding contests and bodybuilders themselves, I have seen this phenomenon over and over again. It may seem the right thing to do at the time, but to tell a bodybuilder that he "looks great on stage, and is definitely going to win" or that "you should have won . . . you're twice as good as the guy who won" is wrong and ultimately cruel (unless of course it happens to be true).

Bodybuilders are not able to see how they *stack up* alongside their competitors. They may look fabulous in the gym or in the bathroom mirror, but on stage is a different story. You are no longer alone. You are accompanied by up to one hundred other guys who also think they have a good enough physique to win the title. When you come out on stage to be compared in the relaxed position by the judges, you should stand straight with your weight evenly distributed on both feet. Keep your lats fairly well spread (not excessively) and your thighs tensed (this is where your practice pays off). One of the most gruelling parts of a contest is during the judging when you have to maintain tensed thigh muscles for the entire period in which you are being viewed by the panel.

Make sure the number you were given is pinned on your trunks in a way that the judges can read it clearly. It is also advisable to memorize the number because you may be called by number to come forward to be compared with another competitor.

During the pre-judging it is a good idea to have a knowledgeable friend in the front row. Someone who can signal you should you not be standing correctly. This person with a slight movement of the hand can tell you to move into a more advantageous position. He or she can tell you to step forward, or backwards to take advantage of the overhead lighting. Perhaps you have forgotten to flex your thighs or abs? Someone in the audience who can secretly communicate with you can be of great help. To my certain knowledge, most top pro bodybuilders competing in the Olympia contest each year get some direction from either their wives, girlfriends or training partners during the pre-judging of the contest. This has been going on for years, yet is never talked about openly.

If you are lucky enough to be selected to pose-off (usually the top six to ten bodybuilders will be invited to pose-off to find out who can outpose, outmuscle who), you must be prepared to fight hard and long. This is definitely no place for the faint-hearted. You must be in condition to pose continually, wrenching every last drop of sweat from your body, for up to five full minutes. At no time should you give in and stop posing, for this may be construed by the

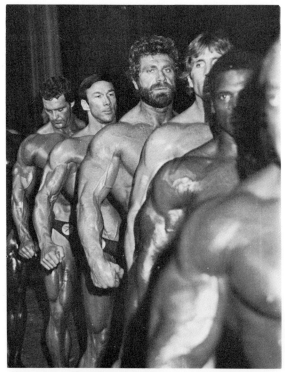

Illus. 273.   The "lineup." Now the show begins.

160

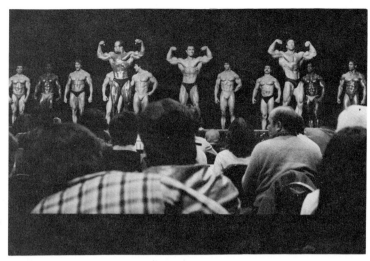

Illus. 274. Competitors are called forward for comparison. Here Beckles, Makkawy and Coe compare arms.

judges as admitting defeat. The aim of a pose-off of course is to show that you have the best body on stage. You need to keep the judges' eyes on you. To pull this off you have to tense and pose nonstop. Be the last to stop posing. You need to show definition, vascularity, size, shape, hardness, and posing originality ad infinitum. . . . The key phrase? "Keep it going!"

Backstage, try to find yourself a quiet corner where you can relax and at least try to keep the usual backstage hustle and bustle out of your mind. But be aware of what is going on: Keep alert as to when you will be called on stage. Some bodybuilders almost hide away backstage. They seek some place where they can lie down and take it easy. Very few competitors can *really* relax backstage, but it is better to try than to pace up and down and involve yourself in the inevitable behind-the-scenes chaos.

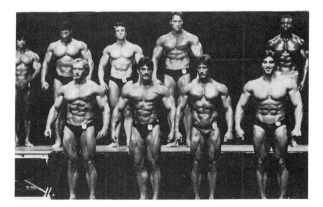

Illus. 275. The day of the show, all competitors are compared in relaxed and posed positions.

At one Mr. Olympia contest (1979, Columbus, Ohio) Frank Zane, the ultimate winner, was nowhere to be found backstage. This caused not a little confusion among the officials and fellow competitors. Later we were to find out that Frank was in the parking lot behind the theatre in a friend's trailer, complete with weights for pumping up. He turned up at the pre-judging pumped and oiled—from "nowhere"—and swept to victory. Even if this tactic didn't clinch the title for Zane, it did help him prepare quietly for the event. Zane is not a great believer in "psyching out" the opposition. He prefers to spend the entire year in progressive preparation for a show, and ultimately turn up as near to perfection as he can be.

On the other hand, Arnold Schwarzenegger proudly admits that psychological warfare is part of his game plan. He opens up his bag of mental tricks when it comes to contest time. Even close friends are subjected to ridicule on or off stage if it will give big Arnold the edge. At the 1980 Olympia in Australia, he claimed that his remark to Mike Mentzer about his never becoming a Mr. Olympia because of his "belly hanging out all over the stage" so angered Mentzer that he couldn't pose properly during the proceedings. I find this a little farfetched. At times Mike forgets to tense his abs, but on that day in Sydney, he could never have been justly described as having a "belly." Nor, in my opinion, would any anger he felt have adversely influenced his posing ability.

A further "trick" of Arnold's was played at the expense of Cuban colossus Sergio Oliva. During the 1970 Mr. Olympia contest in New York City, Arnold and Sergio were posing-off on stage to the shouts

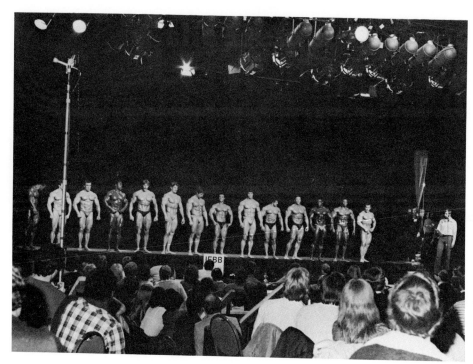

Illus. 276.   An IFBB pro lineup.

and screams of the New York crowd, when at the point of almost total exhaustion Arnold told Sergio, "Let's go," whereupon Sergio, who doesn't have a huge repertoire of poses at the best of times, was happy to step off the plinth to make an offstage exit. Since the crowd was still roaring for more, Arnold shot off several last-minute poses . . . and ultimately, coming to realize what had transpired, wickedly seized the opportunity and actually waved Sergio back to the posing plinth with a gesture that said in no uncertain terms: "What's the matter, Sergio, you scared to pose off with me? Have you chickened out?"

This may have contributed to Arnold's first Olympia win, but it was far more likely due to Arnold's offhand remark to Sergio in Columbus a couple of weeks earlier at the Mr. World contest that he was too skinny and if he hoped to beat him (Arnold) in New York, he had better put on *much* more weight. Sergio had fallen for the bait and quickly added another 10 pounds, which naturally enough

was not all pure muscle, and it had the effect of diminishing Sergio's awesomeness, rather than enhancing it.

The film *Pumping Iron* recorded another cheeky episode, this time involving Lou Ferrigno, of "Incredible Hulk" fame.

Arnold had invited Lou and his father to join him for breakfast the morning of the 1975 Olympia in South Africa. "You look in great shape, Lou!" said Arnold. "But it's such a pity that you didn't have another two weeks to prepare for this show . . .," intimating that Lou wasn't quite "ready" to do battle that morning, at least not with the great Schwarzenegger. "Well . . . too bad," Arnold continued to the then young and inexperienced Ferrigno, "but if you had had two more weeks to get in shape, I too would have had two more weeks, and I would have still been ahead of you!" At this proclamation Ferrigno's mouth dropped open. The psych-out worked. If the two ever met in competition today, the roles in this psyching game could well be reversed.

The California Bodybuilding Scene 30

California! Mention this sun-drenched state to any hardcore bodybuilder and you will immediately grab his complete attention. California is indeed mecca to the ardent dedicated pumper of iron. Everything there is just perfect for him and the weather is simply ideal for training. Rarely does it ever get too hot and even on Christmas day, an iron trainee can build muscle out-of-doors if he wishes to. The climate is so ideal that many of the very top west coast bodybuilding champions have actually finished their first workout by 8 A.M.!

Climate is not the only attractive feature about California. It has more hardcore bodybuilding gyms catering to the advanced muscle man than anywhere else in the world. Hardcore bodybuilding gyms must be clearly distinguished from their health club or spa counterparts shining in all their chrome glory.

The bodybuilder of the 1980s has no use whatsoever for a health club. He demands a hardcore bodybuilding gym simply crammed with heavy training equipment in an atmosphere dedicated to hardcore workouts. A trainee thrives on the positive vibes coming from being in an environment so totally orientated to his main goal: *building muscle!* So for him it *has* to be California, and, in particular, Los Angeles and its surrounding areas.

The California bodybuilding scene has proudly earned its famous reputation in the pages of Joe Weider's *Muscle Builder*, now renamed *Muscle and Fitness* magazine. During the '50s, '60s and '70s,

Weider was mainly responsible for transforming bodybuilding from its humble working class origins into the glamorous and exciting young sport it is today. Names like Reeves, Scott, Ross, Oliva, Draper, and many others became heroes to the true followers of hardcore bodybuilding. Photos and inspiring articles were featured in every single issue of his magazine and you just couldn't wait for the next issue to appear on the newsstands.

Further research into hardcore bodybuilding resulted in astonishing improvements and each new Weider star surpassed the one before him with a far superior physique. New training methods and equipment accounted for the soaring standards of bodybuilding in the last two decades. Vince Gironda, the

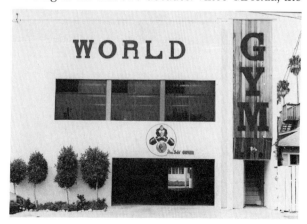

Illus. 277.   Joe Gold's new gym front.

"Iron Guru," pioneered in both areas. During the 1960s Vince boasted that more champions trained at his gym in North Hollywood than anywhere else in the world. Among the most famous were Don Howorth and Larry Scott. The photographs of these two great champions working out together at Vince's gym were truly inspirational the first time they appeared in *Muscle Builder*. It is a gross understatement to say they hit the hardcore bodybuilding audience like a bombshell!

Here for the first time were two of the greatest physiques in the world training on equipment we hadn't even seen before. What was the name of that funny little bench Larry Scott was resting over doing his barbell curls? Why was Howorth using that strange pipelike sliding apparatus for his shoulder presses? Surely this was the birth of modern bodybuilding, refined right then and there in Vince's gym as equipment makers the world over quickly went to their work benches.

One guy with an ingenious talent for building hardcore bodybuilding equipment was Joe Gold, original owner of Gold's Gym. Having first opened his musclebuilding gym way back in 1952 in the jazz capital of New Orleans, Joe eventually got tired of running the gym and sold out. In 1965 he returned to his native California and opened the very first Gold's Gym in Venice Beach. He built the building with his own hands during the day and at night welded the equipment.

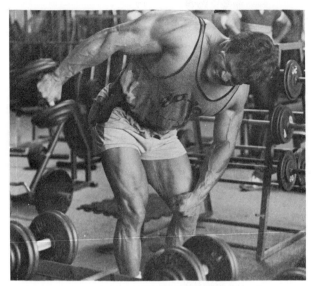
Illus. 279.   Canada's Reid Schindle made the trip to Gold's to train for the Universe competition.

According to Joe, this was just about the first muscle gym ever built catering only to hardcore bodybuilders. So with almost every other gym advertising facilities such as saunas and sun rooms, Joe proudly insisted: "You come to Gold's Gym to *train!* Oh yes, and you can have a shower, too!" Joe Weider took immediate advantage of this new muscle-building emporium and, according to Joe Gold, "sent every one of his new protégés down there to work out and be photographed."

Indeed the building was simply ideal for photography. Having huge glass windows and skylights, the entire hardcore bodybuilding fraternity was once again mesmerized by those fantastic training shots regularly coming out of Gold's in the pages of Joe Weider's muscle journal. Arnold who had been brought to America by Weider now galvanized everyone's attention to Gold's.

Setting up his training camp at Gold's, Arnold joined forces with Frank Zane, Franco Columbu and Dave Draper to prepare for the 1970 NABBA Mr. Universe in London, England. Once again Weider serialized the events and *Muscle Builder* featured the best set of training photographs ever seen at that time, mostly taken by Artie Zeller. Arnold has said many times that he experienced the best workouts of his life, thanks mainly to the atmosphere at Gold's Gym. Not surprisingly, this new Gold's team simply took over the NABBA show. Columbu came in second behind Chris Dickerson and Draper placed third behind Reg Park and Arnold. Frank Zane won the amateur title and of course Arnold won the pro.

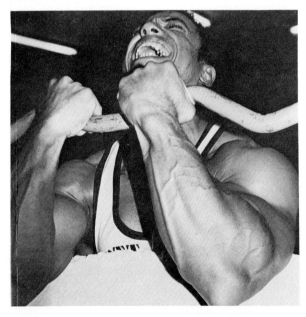
Illus. 278.   Chris Dickerson gives everything on the last rep of Scott curls.

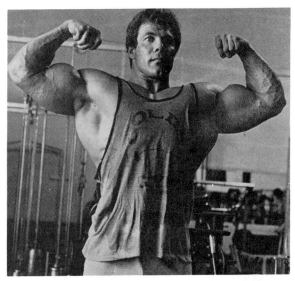

Illus. 280.   *Reid Schindle flexes up after a set of bench presses.*

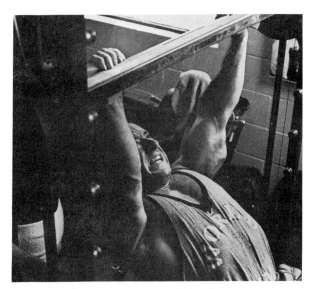

Illus. 281.   *"One more rep, Rocky . . ."*

Arnold said of his life-long hero Reg Park: "Reg cannot hope to get into top shape training in South Africa. He must come to California and Gold's Gym to train along with me and the rest of the champs. Then and only then will he have a chance to beat me!"

In 1970 Joe Gold again became bored. The gym was an enormous financial success, but the spirit in the old sea dog was still unfulfilled, so once again he sold out. After travelling around the world, Joe was quite surprised when he was offered the gym back again five years later by Ken Sprague who had bought it while Joe was away at sea. While Joe was away the gym had been moved from Venice to Main Street right in the heart of Santa Monica. The deal with Sprague never came off, though, and Joe decided he would build another gym. Being unable to call his own gym Gold's because of a contractual agreement, Joe named his new place World Gym and now we had two great hardcore bodybuilding gyms in the L.A. area.

The original Gold's changed hands again. This time Pete Grymkowski, a super-star bodybuilder in his own right, Ed Connors, a successful business man and Tim Kimber took over. Treating the gym in a very professional business-like manner, these three moved Gold's from Santa Monica back to Venice Beach, only one mile from the World Gym.

The gym itself is simply out of this world. Taking up a whole office block it is absolutely crammed with every piece of bodybuilding apparatus imaginable—Nautilus, Corbin Gentry and Universal—all fit

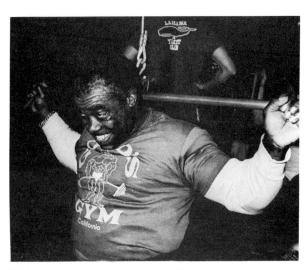

Illus. 282.   *Johnny Fuller works his back.*

snugly among the multitude of pulleys, barbells, dumb-bells and other conventional training equipment. The gym is spotlessly clean and you can always be assured of a warm and friendly greeting each time you visit, no matter what part of the world you come from.

Bodybuilders now have a choice between two different training atmospheres. If you're the type of individual who likes working out to hard rock, you should enjoy Gold's. In fact, many guys actually train at both gyms depending on their mood. Dickerson, Platz, Bannout and Waller, for instance, alternate between them. Yet Arnold and Franco wouldn't even think of training anywhere else but at World.

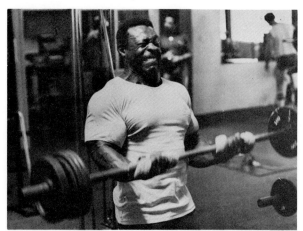

Illus. 283.   Canada's Roy Callender gives his arms a workout.

In early March of 1981 Roy Callender of Montreal, Canada made his pilgrimage to California to prepare for the IFBB California Grand Prix. Roy chose to train at World Gym and when asked why he needed to incur the extra expense of moving to California just to train for a physique contest Roy replied, "You cannot train like you should at home. You have too many distractions. There's your family to think about, your job, and many other problems that are just constantly working against you. When I want to get into the best shape of my life I come to California. There's no place like it. The weather here is so perfect for bodybuilding—you actually *feel* like training every day, something I don't feel like doing back home. With just one change of clothing plus my training gear I intend to do nothing else but train, eat and sleep bodybuilding until the actual day of the contest!"

Roy Callender returned to California once again that year, in August, a full two months before the 1981 IFBB Mr. Olympia. Once again he made the World Gym his training headquarters. Sticking rigidly to a daily ritual of workouts, this famous bodybuilding star appeared in the best condition of his life. In fact, many many people thought that Roy Callender was the one who should have won the 1981 IFBB Mr. Olympia.

Surely he was the most muscular man on stage that day. He was also probably the most muscular man the world had ever seen! "They told me that if ever I came in ripped I should win the 'Olympia'. So I came in ripped. What more can I say?" were Roy's words after the results were announced.

To acquire that unbelievable ripped condition Roy followed a torturous routine that would have killed the average hardcore bodybuilding enthusiast.

Renting a small motel room only walking distance from the World Gym, Roy awoke at 7 A.M. each morning to a breakfast consisting of fifteen hard-boiled egg whites, a 10-ounce dish of plain yoghurt mixed with crushed fresh pineapple, and water. The yolk of the egg was eliminated because of its undesirably high fat content. After his workout Roy once again retired to his lonely motel room for lunch which consisted merely of one and a half pounds of boiled fish or sometimes a pound of turkey, plus a little water. At night Roy simply survived on pieces of lettuce, some nuts and a few seeds!

When confronted with this gruelling spartan diet routine, Roy observed: "Look, if I'm gonna sit down before a meal and say, 'Yuk! This is terrible!' then I might as well go home today. I've never ever dieted so constructively or consistently as this before. I believe that diet is 70 percent of the game and come Olympia time, I'll be ripped!"

Vitamin supplements in very high dosages were also included in Roy's special diet. Being a total believer in vitamin C, Roy used it in an effort to improve muscular recuperation. He consumed 3,000 mg. of this vitamin every single day! Roy enthusiastically endorses vitamin C as ". . . one of the reasons why I can train for fiteen days in a row without becoming overtrained or burned out!" Roy loaded up on desiccated liver tablets too.

When questioned about the obvious imbalance of essential nutrients in this pre-Olympia diet, Roy

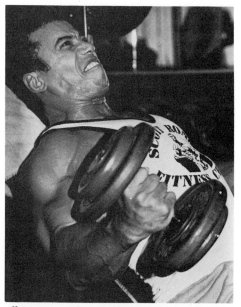

Illus. 284.   Chris Dickerson going all out on incline curls.

166

admitted to occasionally adding a piece of fresh fruit, in spite of hearing that Chris Dickerson would do without even the smallest amount of fruit for a full two months prior to the contest!

Roy insisted he couldn't understand why many young bodybuilders consistently ingested huge amounts of protein in their efforts to build more muscle, and he described the counting of calories or carbohydrates as pure GARBAGE! "Look in the mirror and it will tell you what you have to do!" was Roy's final word on diet.

For those down-hearted hardcore bodybuilders currently plagued by muscular tendon injuries or similar problems, one successful antidote could be the observation of a Roy Callender workout. Training in the most impeccable style, Roy Callender working out is an inspirational sight to behold. Without the slightest degree of heave, sway, or jerk, Roy Callender executes each movement and repetition in the most concentrated, methodical and flawless fashion you could imagine.

Using mind over matter principles, he forces his muscles to handle more stress than the actual poundage attached to the barbell or dumb-bell. This superior ability to focus his entire concentration on the action of the muscle is what separates Roy Callender from the rest of the hardcore brigade. Totally oblivious to all sights and sounds around him, Roy mentally prepares himself to approach the bar for one of his many sets on such a basic exercise as the standing barbell curl.

Placing a piece of sponge in the palm of each hand (a Callender trademark), Roy takes an even, medium-width grip on the barbell. Squeezing the sponge and bar tightly together Roy takes a few deep breaths and then quietly lifts the weight from its resting place on the bench in front of him. Without the slightest degree of body movement, he lifts the bar slowly and curls it right into his neck. The movement is then halted briefly at this contracted position and the biceps muscles are flexed as hard as possible before returning to the starting position.

Roy commenced his first set of basic barbell curls with very moderate poundage for someone of his size and strength. Although most of his sets were performed using a barbell of no more than 100 pounds, Roy often increased his weights when he felt the urge to do so, and sometimes he would work with 120 or 130 pounds. This variation in poundage depended entirely on the responses signalling to him from his biceps. Caring nothing about the amount of weight, repetitions or sets being used, Roy Callender

continued until he felt his biceps had taken all they could, by which time those arm muscles appeared to have doubled in size.

After a short rest from his barbell curls, Roy Callender decided to place the finishing touches on those biceps by shifting concentration to the preacher bench curl. Using a grip of about 3 inches between each hand, Roy did his preacher curls from a base pulley hand-made by Joe Gold himself. Extending his upper arms all the way over the bench so that his armpits came into contact with its top, Roy smoothly pulled on the handle until it reached his chin. He paused slightly in this position, contracting the biceps muscles hard and then slowly returned the weight back to the starting position. After the work done on the barbell curls, it was quite obvious that each rep of the preacher curls was extremely painful as Roy tightly gritted his teeth in an effort to complete rep after rep.

As with the barbell curls, Roy did many sets on the preacher bench until finally he felt he couldn't take any more. Triceps work was next. Unlike many other top champion bodybuilders, Roy did not employ lying barbell extensions, dips or pushdowns for his triceps. He chose two infrequently-used exercises, and the first one was the lying two-dumb-bell extension.

Lying on the bench so that his head was hanging over one end, Roy held two dumb-bells at arm's length above his chest as though he was about to perform bent arm flyes for the chest. With both hands squeezing the sponge covering each dumb-bell handle, Roy now allowed each "bell" to simultaneously be lowered right over his head and as far behind his neck as possible. After a slight pause at the bottom the "bells" were then pushed back to complete lock-out, and those triceps muscles were flexed and contracted as hard as possible. Once again Roy performed the exercise in ultrastrict fashion, allowing his elbows to flair outwards slightly during the course of the movement.

Roy's other triceps exercise was executed on a base pulley. Sitting on a tiny little stool about 18 inches high, Roy attached a short bent triceps bar to the pulley. Sitting with his back to the weight, Roy placed his sponges on each end and with a thumbs-free grip on the handle, slowly lifted it from behind his back to arm's length behind him. From this position Roy allowed the weight to slowly descend as far behind his neck as he possibly could. With teeth-gritting effort Roy now attempted to push the handle back to the starting position for a total muscular

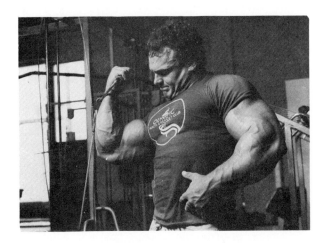

Illus. 285.   Tim Belknap, the sensation of the 80s, sweats it out on cable curls.

contraction of those often hard-to-reach triceps muscles.

In complete contrast to many earlier textbook instructions stating that the triceps extension exercise must be performed with the elbows kept inwards, Roy Callender allowed his upper arms to sway outwards as much as he felt they should—a far safer and less injurious way to perform the exercise.

Thanks to this superhuman regimen, Roy Callender shocked the world at the 1981 Mr. Olympia!

1981 was also the year that the important AAU Mr. America contest would once again be staged at the fabulous venue known as Caesars Palace in Las Vegas, Nevada. That year a young bodybuilder who only three or four months previously had been a virtual unknown was given the edge. Having been featured in regular monthly installments in the pages of Joe Weider's *Muscle and Fitness*, this complete unknown was now literally transformed into a world superstar by the day of the contest. Readers just couldn't believe their own eyes at the sight of this young pocket Hercules weighing a full 220 pounds and sporting 21-inch arms at a height of only 5 feet 4 inches.

Tim Belknap too made his way down to sunny California to train for Mr. America, and for him it just had to be the new Gold's Gym. Arriving at the L.A. International Airport three weeks prior to the contest, Tim bore almost no resemblance to the Tim Belknap who would walk away with that 1981 Mr. America title. Although absolutely massive, Tim appeared pale and quite smooth-looking upon arrival. Surely he couldn't win such a prestigious title as Mr. America . . . or could he?

Unlike Callender, Tim Belknap's pre-Mr. America workouts lasted only about 50 minutes each beginning daily at 3 P.M. Employing huge ponderous weights, Tim displayed the brute strength of a powerlifter while employing the perfect exercise style of a seasoned professional. Although the poundages Tim used were of powerlifting standard, he performed a lot of reps on most of his exercises. It appeared that a guideline of 3 sets of 12 reps was key to Tim Belknap's routine. On paper 3 sets of 12 reps may look like child's play, but not when done the Belknap way.

His exercises were executed in the normal single or orthodox fashion and there was no room for any supersets, tri-sets or compound systems. When you perform 12 reps as intensely as Tim does, then you simply do not have to superset them with any other exercise. Obviously Tim preferred to totally concentrate the whole of his effort into that one particular movement, milking every drop out of it!

Whereas Callender chose to move the bar under total control and concentration at all times, Tim Belknap used immense strength and power to propel his poundages while not sacrificing sharp concentration and strict exercise form. Three sets of 12 reps on the incline curl exercise using two 80-pound dumb-bells requires exceptional concentration and immense superstrength!

During the three-week period he was stationed in California, Belknap literally transformed himself. Even Gold's Gym owner Pete Grymkowski, who at first was not particularly impressed with Tim when he first arrived, was totally flabbergasted at the Mr.

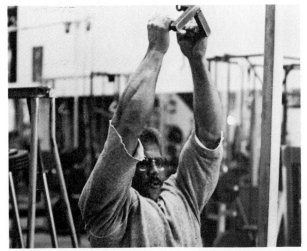

Illus. 286.   Pete Grymkowski, owner of the fabulous Gold's Gym in Venice, California, takes some of his own medicine.

America contest. The three main ingredients in Tim Belknap's amazing three-week transformation were a beautiful deep California suntan, a fish and water diet and intense workouts at Gold's Gym. Nothing beats a good deep suntan when it comes to that finished contest look. Tim who had arrived in California looking quite pale by contest day had the best golden brown suntan of any competitor which made his appearance all the more stunning. Without an ounce of fat on him this totally natural suntan made him stand out relaxed in the lineup.

It seems that fish, chicken and turkey are in and red meat (steaks, beef, etc.) are definitely out when it comes to the pre-contest diet. Hardcore bodybuilders of the past feasted on endless steaks but their modern 1980s counterparts must shun these treats, if they want to achieve that "ultraripped" look.

Tim Belknap at the '81 Mr. America was easily the most ripped and massively muscular Mr. America of all time! Tim's diet played a major part in that look. Allowing himself only one tin of water-packed tuna fish about an hour prior to his afternoon workout, Tim proved how dedicated and disciplined he could be once he set his mind upon that Mr. America goal.

Tim is a diabetic which certainly didn't help him during those last few torturous days before the contest as his body weight dropped several pounds to 198 and his craving for energy foods became almost unbearable.

Tim Belknap stated that when in California he wouldn't dream of training anywhere else but Gold's Gym. For him the boisterous and exciting atmosphere of Gold's was the only way to go. Following a three-day-split routine, Tim worked chest and back one day, legs the next, and shoulders and arms on the third day. Tim was observed at Gold's going through a very simple but very effective and intense arm routine which consisted of:

1. Standing barbell curls 3 sets, approximately 12 reps

2. Incline dumb-bell curls 3 sets, approximately 12 reps

3. One-arm base pulley curls 2 sets, approximately 12 reps

4. Lying triceps extensions 3 sets, approximately 12 reps

5. Triceps pushdowns 3 sets, approximately 12 reps

6. Close-grip bench presses 3 sets, approximately 12 reps

Using brutal poundages on the standing barbell curl, Tim worked until the bar almost fell out of his hands! Three sets of at least 12 repetitions on the incline dumb-bell curl with 75- and 80-pound dumb-bells are an incredible feat for any bodybuilder, let alone for Tim Belknap who has been training only five years!

When Tim demonstrated the one-arm base pulley curl, every arm muscle in his body appeared to be near bursting point as he accented the movement. Two sets to absolute muscular failure on this one after the very heavy proceeding barbell and dumb-bell work felt like the icing on the cake! Adding up the poundage on the exercise bar which Tim selected for his lying triceps extensions quickly revealed that it held more than most semi-advanced bodybuilders used for their *bench press!* Maybe that's why he has 21-inch arms.

Triceps pushdowns were performed using a width grip of at least 18 inches between his hands and a thumbs-free "false grip," completely contracting his triceps muscles as hard as he could at the bottom position of the movement. When his triceps were totally exhausted from these extensions and pushdowns, Tim finished them off completely with 3 sets of 12 reps on the close-grip bench press movement, taking full advantage of the unused strength and power inside his larger, more powerful chest and shoulder muscles. The workout itself was carried out at a fairly brisk pace and Tim wasted no time at all in going from set to set and exercise to exercise as soon as his breath had returned to normal.

Three weeks later Tim Belknap was crowned 1981 AAU Mr. America!

"Early to bed, early to rise" is a "muscle motto" high on the list of Bronston Austin's precontest training preparation. When in hard training for a show or exhibition Bronston rises at 5:30 A.M. each day and drives from Los Angeles to Santa Monica for his daily ritual of muscle building. Arriving at the World Gym just before 7 A.M., Bronston prepares his body for its daily bombardment of exercise. Being absolutely convinced that the body must be kept constantly warm throughout the workout, he covers himself from head to toe in a muscle rub lotion. Placing a rubber slimming belt over his waist and hips, Bronston slips on his training suit and gloves, and is ready to hit the weights.

Bronston is an emphatic believer in training only one body part, one set of muscles at a workout. In this way he can be sure he is giving a muscle group his whole attention. After a brief warm-up

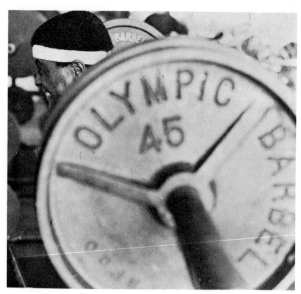

Illus. 287. Bronston Austin squatting.

consisting of light stretching exercises, Bronston prepares to spend the next two hours training only his chest! Taking several minutes to psych himself up for each set, Bronston Austin has a very methodical, precise and smooth training style that is inspiring to behold.

Bronston's first exercise is lying bent-arm pullovers for the rib cage. Lying on a very low exercise bench, Bronston holds the barbell across his lower chest. His hands are spaced about 15 to 18 inches apart and from this position he allows the bar to travel right over his face and down to near the floor. In this position he gives his rib cage a terrific stretch. He works the exercise until he cannot do another set in strict style and at one point it looks as though his eyes are coming out of his head as he tries desperately to force out those reps.

After 6 sets of pullovers Bronston moves into his second exercise: Wrapping his hands around a short rope which is attached to the lat machine, Bronston kneels on the gym floor with his thighs spread well apart. Holding the rope so that his palms are facing away from him, Bronston pulls the rope and his upper body down to the floor. Just before he reaches the floor he rotates both wrists so that his palms are now facing him. In the completed position Bronston's elbows are in contact with his knees and his forehead is now actually touching his hands. This type of pulldown when performed in the manner described is simply unbeatable for developing those hard-to-reach finger-like muscles known as the *serratus*.

Bronston does each set in a very slow, calculated fashion, also mentally contracting his *serratus* muscles at the contracted position. He does 6 sets of 15 reps on these pulldowns and then makes his way over to the bench press. Bronston starts fairly light on this one, working up to extremely heavy weights. His smooth methodical training style is very similar to Callender's, but on the bench press he deliberately adds on much heavier weights each set until his goals for the exercise are met. Selecting a thumbs-free false grip on the barbell, Bronston placed his sweat towel across his chest while performing the movement. He allows the bar to just graze the towel each time and then he thrusts it back to arm's length again.

Following about 8 to 10 pound increments each set, Bronston now makes his way over to the sliding incline press device which is positioned in the corner of the room. The incline angle of about 70° to 75° chosen for this exercise is decidedly more severe than is commonly used. Bronston positions himself so that both elbows will travel way back each time the bar comes in contact with his neck. As with the bench press, Bronston uses a "false" grip on the bar and increases his poundages each set.

Next on the agenda are lying dumb-bell bent-arm flyes. After maybe two warm-up sets on the flyes, Bronston stays with a pair of 60-pound dumb-bells for his next 6 soul-inspiring sets of this exercise. Lying with his upper body on the bench he holds the "sixties" above his chest with both palms facing each other. Keeping his arms bent throughout the entire movement, Bronston allows them to travel outwards as far as he possibly can. In this position he appears to be mentally concentrating and stretching his pectoral muscles to their maximum. As Bronston pushes himself to do more and more reps, his tendons and neck muscles seem like they might burst right through the skin as he pushes himself through the pain barrier.

Although quite capable of handling much heavier weights, Bronston demonstrates one of the very few secrets to successful hardcore bodybuilding progress, namely, "Always keep your weights under total control!"

Using the same pair of sixties, Bronston now moves over to another incline bench set to a 75° angle and continues the onslaught to his upper pectoral muscles. Performing incline dumb-bell bent-arm flyes, he amazingly allows the bells to travel as far outwards as he can and it looks as though his pecs might be ripped right out of their sockets!

When it seems that he might not be capable of completing another full rep, Bronston cleverly changes the exercise into a strict incline pressing movement using the strength and power of his triceps muscles. He is really beginning to feel things now and each set sees him constantly gritting his teeth as he fights like mad to complete his repetitions. He does so many sets of this exercise that his light grey training suit is now dyed almost black with sweat.

Without too much rest Bronston goes into his next chest exercise which is cable pulley crossovers. From the arms-outstretched position, he "leans" into the movement as he allows one arm to cross over the other at the contracted point in the exercise. He does a total of 8 sets on this exercise for about 12 to 15 reps per set.

Wide-grip parallel bar dips are next and Bronston does these wearing a harness around his neck from which a 30-pound dumb-bell is strapped. Dipping as low as he possibly can, Bronston appears to be in terrific pain as he pushes his pectoral muscles nearer and nearer to the ground. After six gruelling sets of these, Bronston now reaches his ninth and final direct chest exercise which are pec squeezes on the pec deck.

He uses even more mental concentration on this movement and as he sits there grasping onto the pads of the machine you can hear him breathing deeply in and out. Selecting such a heavy poundage on the machine that it requires him to actually lift his body right out of the seat, he finds himself struggling after only 6 to 8 reps. Bronston continually pushes himself to absolute muscular failure, or until he cannot squeeze the pads together any longer. Six sets on the pec deck mean the end of Bronston Austin's chest routine, and an even longer drive back home.

Illus. 288.   Thigh curling—but check the arms.

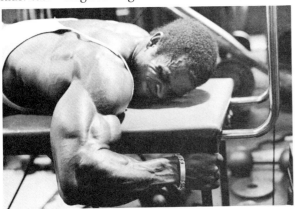

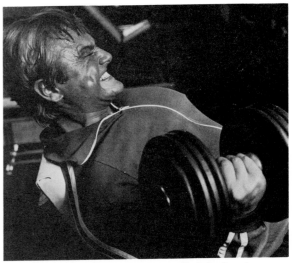

Illus. 289.   Tom Platz has been called the hardest trainer of them all.

Reid Schindle, the massive athlete from Canada was another hardcore bodybuilder who made California his temporary home while preparing for the 1981 Mr. Canada title. Setting up his training headquarters at Gold's, Reid religiously trained twice every day on a double-split routine in an effort to get his body ripped in time for the contest. Rising at 7 A.M. each day and breakfasting on only black coffee and half a cantaloupe, Reid was in Gold's just after 8:30 A.M. He was regularly observed performing a great many supersets and compound sets.

Employing a system of at least 20 sets per body part, Reid would group two exercises together for one particular body part. He would do as many reps as he felt were necessary and then move right into the second exercise. Five of these circuit-type sequences would be completed before grouping together another two direct exercises for that individual muscle group. Like Bronston Austin, Reid preferred to concentrate on only one particular body part each time he trained, but he didn't believe in the "training to total failure" philosophy. Reid felt that kind of system was far too severe and he couldn't make the kind of gains he wanted from this high-intensity, low-sets principle.

One particular exercise Reid used to build his huge back was the seated "V" Bar pulldown to the chest. Seated on a special low stool rigged up at Gold's, Reid inserted both hands into the "V"-shaped handles attached to the pulley and with the strength and power of his upper back muscles, pulled hard on them until they reached his upper chest. Reid used tremendously heavy poundages on this exercise

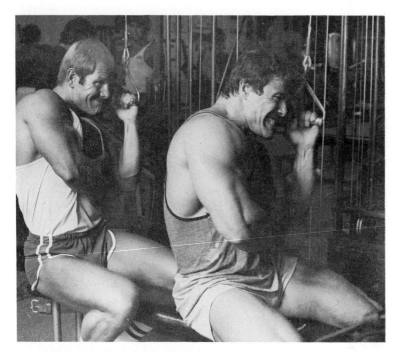

Illus. 290.   Reid Schindle and partner work special "serratus" pulley in unison.

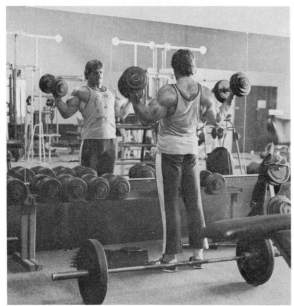

Illus. 291.   Super-conditioned natural bodybuilder Rod Koontz trains biceps.

which meant he had to lower himself backwards until his upper body was almost parallel to the floor! Performing pulldowns in this manner was only possible because of the T–bar which secured his legs and body, preventing them from being raised off the floor. Reid was able to achieve a terrific contraction of his back muscles from this exercise and he alter-nated it set for set with the regular lat machine pulldown behind the neck.

Another novel and unique exercise used by Reid in an effort to bring out the serratus and intercostal muscles was the one arm seated twisting pulldown on the lat machine. On this one, Reid and his training partner performed the exercise simultaneously. Straddled across the exercise bench they worked the left side of their bodies first. Grabbing hold of a handle attached to the pulley with his left hand, Reid twisted his wrist in a corkscrew fashion as he pulled the handle as far down as he could. The repetitions were performed at a very fast speed and they both quickly knocked out 5 sets of 20 to 30 reps for each side of their bodies.

Time out for lunch which consisted of fresh fish baked over a charcoal fire, fresh tossed salad and a little water. Sunbathing after lunch, Reid returned to Gold's at 5 P.M. for his second workout of the day. Dinner at 8 P.M. would consist only of fresh turkey and a little salad. He would then retire for the night and repeat the process the following day.

On September 15, Reid Schindle won his fifth Mr. Canada title!

While it has been noted that the stars of the hardcore bodybuilding world have made California their temporary home in order to prepare for an important show or contest, some of these great champions have actually moved out there for good! One champion who made the permanent move to California is "Mr. Heavy Duty," Mike Mentzer. Living in Palm Springs, Mike still travels two or three times a week to Gold's Gym for the sole purpose of savagely attacking those heavy-duty Nautilus machines.

Insisting that the heavy duty principles of modern day hardcore bodybuilding are the best, Mike can regularly be seen utilizing these methods on such machines as the Nautilus biceps machine, the Nautilus shrug machine and many other ingenious devices capable of standing up to his demanding training methods.

Greg "Rocky" De Ferro and his new wife Karen can be seen working out together at the World Gym on a three-day split routine cycle followed by a full day's rest and Rocky can also be observed receiving forced reps from Karen when he finds himself unable to complete another full rep on his own. He can count on Karen always being on hand to assist him with the bar when he runs into difficulty.

With more and more famous champion bodybuilders such as Bertil Fox, Tom Platz, Chris Dickerson and Samir Bannout regularly migrating to sunny California, it's now becoming more common for the truly dedicated hardcore bodybuilder to at least visit the scene, even as an observer. He won't be disappointed in what he finds.

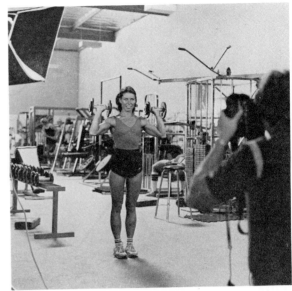

Illus. 292.   *Lyn Conkwright demonstrates women's weight training for the cameras of* Muscle and Fitness.

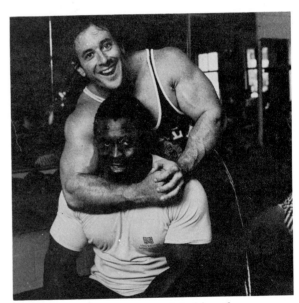

Illus. 293.   *Rocky puts a stranglehold on the formidable Roy Callender.*

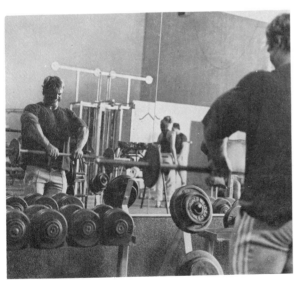

Illus. 294.   *Note the way Tom Platz holds the upright row bar forward during the exercise.*

A History of the Bench Press 31

The most popular weight-training exercise is undoubtedly the bench press. It is a key part of the routines of bodybuilders, powerlifters and athletes, and even people not familiar with weight training are aware of the bench press. To many people, the amount of weight one can lift in the bench press is an indication of one's strength.

The bench press is one of the three competition powerlifts virtually every bodybuilder includes in his routine, and for many it is the key chest exercise. The explosion of women's bodybuilding and powerlifting has increased the market for bench press performers substantially.

On a more personal level, the bench press flour-

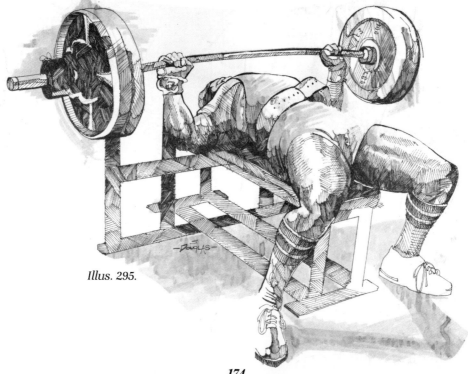

Illus. 295.

ishes because it appeals to our inherent laziness. It allows us to lie on our backs and be very comfortable during its performance. It also appeals to our narcissism in that it develops the showy shoulder and chest muscles of the upper torso. Finally, it appeals to our ego in that heavy weights can be handled. In fact, more weight can be lifted in the bench press than in any other upper body exercise.

The bench press hasn't always been the weightman's favorite. It wasn't until the 1950s that people became aware of its benefits and its popularity began to grow, displacing the standing press as the preferred upper body exercise. The first person to really popularize the bench press was Vancouver strongman Doug Hepburn. Although an excellent Olympic lifter (world heavyweight champion in 1953), he enjoyed doing other lifts, particularly the bench press. Doug's best bench press was 580 pounds while weighing 270. Had there been formal competition on a regular basis in Hepburn's day, it's probably a safe bet to say that he would have been the first to reach 600 pounds.

About the same time in New York City, Marvin Eder, an outstanding Olympic lifter and bodybuilder, placed third in the 1951 Mr. America contest. Eder was naturally suited for the bench press. Using a wide collar-to-collar grip, he benched 510 pounds while weighing 200. Using a regulation grip he did 485 and even more amazing was his ability to perform a dip with 435 additional pounds. If nothing else, this should show the importance of performing dips as an assistance exercise for the bench press.

Although best known for his squatting ability (he's done 1200 pounds) former Olympic champion Paul Anderson was also an excellent bench presser. Despite never really specializing in the lift, he was

Illus. 296.   Big Jim Williams unofficially bench-pressing 705 lbs in practice at York Barbell Club.

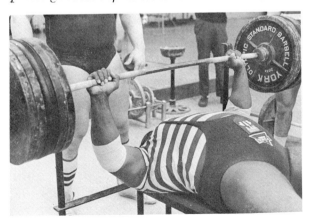

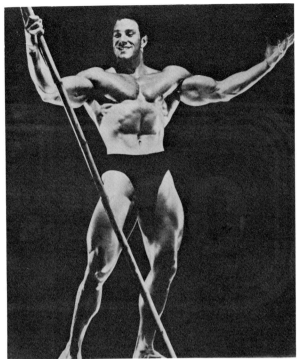

Illus. 297.   Reg Park is one of the first men to bench press 500 lbs.

reported to have raised 627 pounds as a professional. This would make him the first person to break the 600-pound barrier.

By the late 1950s the bench press came of age. As in other areas of bodybuilding, California was the trendsetter in popularizing the bench press. Probably the best known Californian was Pat Casey. Pat Casey's first claim to fame came during the 1957 Teenage Mr. America contest in San Francisco where he startled the judges by telling them he could bench 420. One of the judges at the contest was four-time Mr. Universe, Bill Pearl. Bill was so impressed with Pat that he asked him for advice and corresponded with him regularly. Pat eventually joined Bill's gym in Los Angeles and became the first person to officially break the 600-pound barrier when he benched 617¼ in 1967. In practice he was reported to have lifted 640.

Two other outstanding Californians were Chuck Ahrens and Steve Marjanian, both of Los Angeles. Ahrens was the mystery man of the bodybuilding and lifting world. He rarely, if ever, trained his legs, preferring to concentrate on his upper body. Also, it was reported that he was never seen with his shirt off. There is, however, in existence a picture of him rolling up his sleeve and revealing a monstrous 23-inch upper arm. Ahrens had incredible arm and

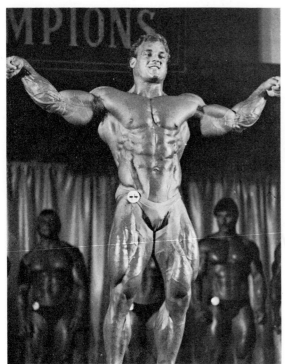

Illus. 298.   Muscle phenomenon Tim Belknap does 385 for 10 reps as part of his regular training.

Illus. 299.   Pat Neve is a former power lifter with incredible bench-pressing power.

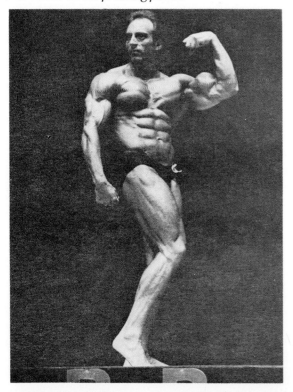

shoulder strength and one of his best lifts was the bench press, in which he had raised at least 565. He was reported on one occasion to have benched 400 pounds 28 times in succession. Although highly unlikely, it does make you wonder about his super-strength.

Marjanian, like Ahrens, did little work for his legs, preferring to concentrate on his chest and shoulders. Although his best lift was the seated behind-the-neck press, he once hoisted 315 pounds for 5 reps and also excelled at the bench press, capably heaving an easy 500 pounds.

A transplanted Californian by way of Sweden, Karl Norberg was an inspiration to older men everywhere. In characteristic style with his legs high off the bench, Norberg benched an almost unbelievable 460 pounds at the age of 73! Even more amazing was the fact that he didn't *begin* regular weight training until he was in his fifties.

At the other end of the age spectrum were a trio of teenage supermen, Steve Kojigian, Dennis Melke and Rick Giofu. Kojigian was one of the premier bench pressers of the '60s, regardless of age or weight. While only 18 years of age and weighing 181, he benched 450. He later decided to devote himself to the family business. Had he continued to train on a regular basis he might have set records that would still be standing today. Melke was a well-proportioned bodybuilder from Burbank who at the age of 18 could bench 440 while weighing 215. Rick Giofu, who hailed from Detroit, may have been the best of the three. At the mere age of 15 he bench pressed 400 while weighing just over 200. Rick still continues to train, but it's in wheelchair competition. An unfortunate accident left him paralyzed from the waist down.

Bodybuilders have done as much and perhaps more than powerlifters to make the bench press popular. Although many bodybuilders shy away from extremely heavy weights or perform the exercise in such a way that it's difficult to use heavy weights, there are several who are extremely strong in the bench press.

Three-time Mr. Universe Reg Park was capable of benching 520, while Mr. World, Chuck Sipes, could handle 570. Mr. U.S.A., Pat Neve, once held the world record in the 181-pound class with a lift of 468¾. Other bodybuilders who have excelled at the bench press are Franco Columbu who has done 500 and Boyer Coe who benched 420 at the age of 17. The current Mr. America, Tim Belknap, can do 385 pounds for 10 nonlock reps as part of a workout. The list of bodybuilders who are outstanding bench pressers is endless. It makes one wonder how much some of these bodybuilders could bench if they decided to concentrate on the lift.

Athletes, especially football players, have also helped popularize the bench press. At first, weight training was frowned upon because it was believed to make you muscle bound and inhibit performance. Gradually this was disproved and today every professional and most college teams have strength coaches. The two players most responsible for the weight-training revolution among football players were Jack Stroud, a lineman for the New York Giants, and former Heisman Trophy winner, Billy Cannon.

Weight training is so prevalent in the professional ranks that in 1980 a "Strongest Man In Pro Football" contest was held in Auburn, Alabama. The overall winner and best bench presser was Mike Webster of the Pittsburgh Steelers who performed 15 reps with 350 pounds. On the collegiate level, the National Strength Coaches Association has selected an All-American Strength Team for the last three years. The best bench presser on the 1980 team was Dock Luckie, a 261-pound defensive tackle from Florida who has lifted 600. It wasn't a competition lift, but nonetheless it's still a remarkable performance.

By the 1970s powerlifting competitions were being held on a regular basis, and records were being broken almost daily. The most amazing record was set by Jim Williams. During the 1972 World Powerlifting Championships the super heavyweight from Scranton, Pennsylvania, benched a phenomenal 675 pounds. Had he not been forced to withdraw from competition because of personal problems, it's a sure bet that he would have been the first to officially bench 700, a lift that he had done in practice.

Without a doubt the most versatile bench presser of all time is Mike MacDonald. At one time Mike held the record in the 181, 198, 220 and 242 pound classes. When Mike Bridges broke his record in the 181 class, Mike proceeded to break the record in the 242-pound class with a lift of 608 pounds, once again enabling him to hold the record in four different weight classes. As Mike continues to go up in body weight, look for him as a definite promise to be the first person to break the 700-pound barrier.

Other 600-plus benchers during the '70s were Don Reinhoudt, Wayne Bouvier, Lars Hedlund and Bill Kazmaier. Of this group, Hedlund and Kazmaier were clearly the best, both having the potential of

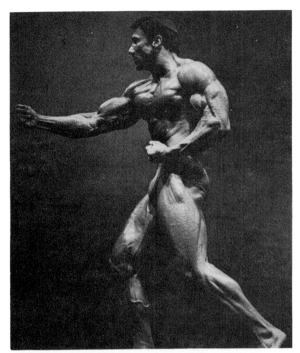

Illus. 300. Boyer Coe—an extremely competitive bodybuilder and a man who could bench press enormous poundage even when only a teenager.

benching 700 pounds. Kazmaier currently holds the world record in the bench press with a lift of 661 pounds (Williams' 675 is considered an American record because world records were not kept until 1973), and did an even more amazing 600 pounds for 5 reps during a meet in Texas in February 1981. Hedlund's chances for 700, however, are a bit dim as he's recovering from an injury. Before the injury, however, he benched 700 in practice and did 600 for 10 reps in a very loose touch-and-go style.

By now many of you are probably thinking that the bench press is the exclusive domain of the big guys. The lighter weight classes, too, have had their share of outstanding bench pressers. Former Olympic lifter Chuck Vinci benched 325 weighing 123 pounds back in 1955. Moving to the present, Joe Bradley in the 132-pound class has done a triple-body weight bench press with 397. Chuckie Dunbar of the 114-pound class has done 314, while the world's greatest powerlifter, Mike Bridges, holds the world record in the 181-pound class with a lift of 529 pounds.

A few years ago, a commercial for a women's cigarette proclaimed, "You've Come a Long Way, Baby." This could also be an accurate description of women's powerlifting and bodybuilding. No longer

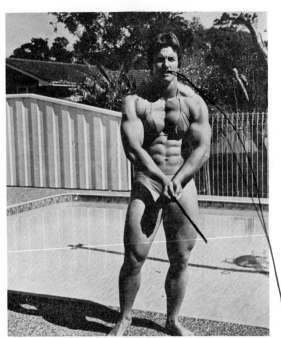

do they train with petite dumb-bells and try to look cute because bodybuilding was considered un-feminine. They're as tough as the guys and handle poundages that would put many of the men to shame. And more women are incorporating body-building exercises into their general fitness routines.

At the 1981 Women's World Powerlifting Championships, Bev Francis of Australia, lifting in the 181-pound class, benched an incredible 330 pounds. When you compare this to the fact that the third-place finisher in the first (1965) Men's Senior National Powerlifting Championships for the 181-pound class benched only 10 pounds more than Ms. Francis, it really becomes obvious how far women have come.

As to the future of the bench press, look for many interesting things to happen. The first official 700-pound bench press should become a reality soon and the gap between men's and women's records should narrow. But most importantly, the bench press will remain the exercise of choice for many.

Illus. 301.   Australia's Bev Francis was the first woman to bench press 300 lbs. She has officially benched 330.

COME ON KIDS! YOU HAVE TO FOLLOW MY BEAT MORE CAREFULLY!

Appendix: Questions and Answers 32

Can you give me an exercise for building the outerhead of the triceps because I lack development in this area? The only equipment I have is a set of barbells and dumb-bells, an E-Z curl bar and an adjustable bench.

The best exercise for the outerhead of the triceps is the supine triceps extension done with a light dumb-bell. Lie on your back on a bench and hold a single dumb-bell at arm's length with your thumb facing downwards until the top of the dumb-bell touches the left pectoral. Return to straight-arm position without any bounce from the chest. Do not use excessive weight which can defeat the purpose of the exercise.

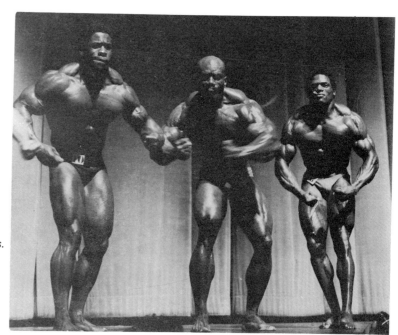

Illus. 302.   Bertil Fox, Sergio Oliva and Tony Pearson in one of the most memorable posedowns of recent times.

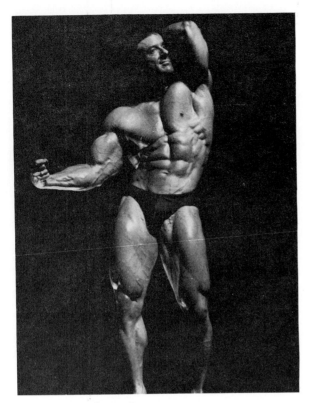

Illus. 303.   *Rocky De Ferro.*

With the pre-exhaust system, after you've done your isolation movement, could you use two combination movements in superset fashion, so as to hit the muscle at different angles?

No! It would be better to use *two* sets to really tire the smaller muscle, and then follow immediately with just one set of a compound movement.

I am six feet tall, 118 pounds, have a long scraggly neck, no traps and my clavicles angle up at about 30° even when I try to force my shoulders down. Please give me the two best trap-building exercises.

The best trap exercises are high pulls from the floor and heavy shrugs. Your clavicle structure indicates that you are predominately ectomorphic. Bodybuilding will help you gain muscular weight, but you will never win Mr. Olympia. You are probably more suited to long-distance running.

I have heard that vitamins can help hemorrhoids. Could heavy squats have caused these?

Possibly, but most hemorrhoids (or piles) are caused by straining which can be the result of constipation. Several studies indicate that the bioflavonoids found in foods rich in Vitamin C may help both hemorrhoids and varicose veins in the legs. An increase of fibre in the diet should help. Consult a physician.

Can a normal woman increase the size of her breasts by the use of weight training or any other form of exercise?

No!

I am having trouble developing the inner head of the triceps, the area nearest the back when the arm is hanging straight down. I use lying extensions, standing dumb-bell extensions and kickbacks.

The best exercise for the inner head of the triceps is the lying triceps stretch, slightly bouncing the weight behind the head on the bench. Quickly follow this with the close-grip bench press, 4 sets of 10 each. No rest between sets. This pre-exhaust technique *works*.

You wrote an article once stating a person with a small chest shouldn't do bench presses, but you didn't say what to use instead.

Perform 6 sets of 8 reps of bent-arm laterals on a 35° bench.

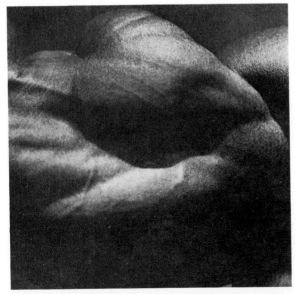

Illus. 304.   *This amazing biceps belongs to Al Beckles.*

I just want to build my upper arms; the rest of my body is all right. Please give me the best exercise to do this.

You are jumping to the erroneous conclusion that there *is* one best exercise to build your arms. The arm has both a pulling and a pushing motion and you need two distinctly different exercises to build both the biceps and the triceps. I suggest you perform 5 sets of 8 reps with the seated dumb-bell curl and 5 sets of 10 reps with the lying triceps stretch. Do both exercises at the same workout and train only every other day. Incidentally, although you will add strength and size to your arms after six weeks on this program, you would make far better progress if you did a complete workout including exercises for *all* the other body parts such as presses, squats, rowing, sit-ups, calf raises and bench presses. One-sided training is never very gratifying.

I have tried heavy-duty training and cannot stay with it for more than a few weeks. I make gains in strength and size and then it all stops; I get fed up and want to quit.

Heavy-duty training (the art of severely limiting sets and increasing all-out intensity) has proven to be very beneficial to some trainers. My advice is to intersperse your heavy-duty training periods with what I call the "Wankers" routine (a British term which will be well understood by my English readers). In other words, take it easy—go in for loads of sets, with less weight, less intensity and less strain. The change could even help growth. Less intense training will allow minor injuries to heal, make for a more relaxed nervous system (too much heavy-duty work on the nerves can upset the body) and generally ready your body for a new onslaught of muscle tendon and strength-building heavy-duty training. I recommend a form of reduced training intensity for the time being to allow your body to recoup; then you can go back to an all-out intensity cycle later on.

I train hard four days a week, but I have a problem with definition. I have cut calories drastically and ingest fewer than my body uses up, but still do not have good definition. My diet includes ham, eggs, bacon, cheeses, sauerkraut and poultry. My only "indulgence" is a penchant for pickles.

You do not say whether you eat fresh fruit and leafy green vegetables. I would feel happier too if

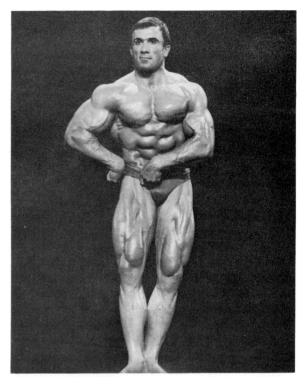

Illus. 305.   Ali Malla.

you included fish in your diet. There are a lot of processed and treated foods in your diet. Ham, bacon, sauerkraut and *particularly* pickles are all very salty which tends to bloat you. Cut them down to a minimum or out altogether.

This hidden salt prevents your diet from working. Nature supplies adequate salt in fruits and vegetables, so stay clear of all foods that have this extra hidden salt and add no salt at the table. Within two weeks you will find your body becoming more defined than ever before.

Can I gain muscle size as quickly using around 15 reps as I could using about 6 reps? Surely it doesn't matter that much because I will still keep adding weight as I get stronger irrespective of how many reps I do.

Generally speaking, higher reps are only suited to those who already have large muscles. Most bodybuilders gain their *initial* size from a system using 6 to 10 reps. Once you have developed a degree of muscle density, you may find that further growth comes quicker from using about 12 reps.

Your argument of being able to increase the weight using any system of reps, although the-

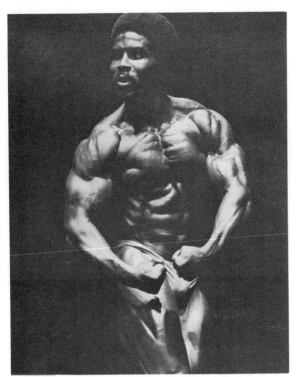

Illus. 306.   Robby Robinson, the Florida-born superstar.

oretically true, does not work out in practice. Otherwise you would get power and Olympic lifters would use sets of high reps to increase strength. Ninety-nine percent of bodybuilders obtain most of their size using repetitions in the medium range, e.g., 6 to 10 reps.

When should someone change one's training routine?

There is no cut-and-dried single answer. It varies from individual to individual. Vince Gironda believes you should "change your routine every three days to avoid staleness." Oscar Heidenstam thinks a change in routine every eight weeks or so is beneficial. Physical culture writer Denie told me that one of the reasons many men make it is because they stick to the exercises that work for them year in and year out. And Steve Reeves reportedly never did the same workout twice.

I can offer you some sound general "ball park" advice:

Beginners to bodybuilding should keep to basic routines for at least three to six months and then only change a few exercises to break up the monotony.

Intermediates should change their routines or

at least 20 percent of their exercises every eight to ten weeks.

Advanced bodybuilders should make whatever changes are necessary to drum up a pump, and if this means changing their respective routines every few days, that is what must be done.

What happens when one gives up bodybuilding training? Will all my muscles suddenly run to fat?

What usually happens is that your muscles will lose some tone and certainly some size. The harder you have worked for your muscles, the quicker they will lose size when you stop training. Contrary to popular opinion, training with heavy weights instead of moderate weights does not mean you will lose muscle size less quickly when you cease training. If you consistently overeat when not training (i.e., continue to ingest many more calories than you expend in energy), the muscles can lose size while the body's fat content increases.

It is more likely that you would lose weight rather than gain it when you cease training, but basically it depends on two things:

1. Your disposition towards weight: If you are inclined to be fat, you may get heavier; If you are inclined to be thin, you will lose.

2. Your level of activity in relation to food intake: overeat and remain inactive and you will gain; undereat while staying active and you will lose weight. Very few bodybuilders cease all forms of physical exercise. They may let up on their training or change to another sport or physical activity. They become bodybuilders in the first place because they couldn't stand inactivity.

I have access to a chin bar and a lat machine, but I do not have time (or energy) to use both. Which is the best apparatus to use for wide lat development?

Each has a unique use. More tensile strength and nervous energy is used in chinning, but make sure you keep the elbows back throughout the entire movement. Most top bodybuilders regularly perform wide-grip chins and there is a definite "look" about the back of a regular wide-grip chinner. On the other hand, the pulldown on the lat machine, if not quite as severe a movement, is more complete in requiring less than body weight to pull the bar down to the sternum or below, something which very few bodybuilders can do on the chin bar because they lack the strength.

Of these two movements that most top bodybuilders find extremely beneficial, I would advise you to go with the chins, but not to discount the lat machine. When you have more time, you could add a few sets to supplement your back training.

My problem is my knees. I am 38 years old and have been training since I was 17. I squat with my heels raised on a 4-inch block, but only use 220 pounds for 5 sets of 10 reps. The only other exercise I do is the leg extension, 5 sets of 6 reps (220 pounds). My knees give me a great deal of pain and seem to be very weak. Sometimes (usually the day after my leg workout), I can hardly walk upstairs and have difficulty squatting even without a weight. Everyday occurrences like getting out of bed present a problem. My thighs are, and have always been, underdeveloped, so I need plenty of regular leg work but what can I do to stop this nagging knee trouble?

Knees can be damaged and painful if you work your legs incorrectly. Some individuals, especially youngsters, can get away with almost any type of heavy leg movement without harm. Others, because of inherited factors or advancing years, have to carefully tailor their leg work to avoid harming the knee area and to adequately stimulate continued gains in strength and development.

Because you are approaching forty, you should thoroughly warm up your knee area with three light sets of 30 reps in the thigh extension exercises. Start the motion slowly; do not kick the weight up. Also, I believe the 4-inch block you are using is too high. Try reducing this height to 2½ inches. Remember to squat down only until the top line of your thighs is parallel to the floor. Under no circumstances do full squats, and needless to say, you should never "bounce" out of a squat.

I strongly suggest that you do no fewer than 15 reps for any leg exercise and always use as nearly perfect exercise form as you can: no kicking, bouncing or cheating. If stricter training and extensive warm-ups do not improve your condition, I suggest you consult your doctor.

Does sunlight aid bodybuilding in any way?
According to Dr. Joseph Meites, Professor of Physiology at Michigan State University, sunlight sets off a series of nervous system chain reactions which result in higher hormone levels. This could benefit the bodybuilder. Lack of adequate sunlight will definitely inhibit your gains. On the other hand, if you lie in the sun too long, you could drastically dissipate your energy to the extent that you couldn't

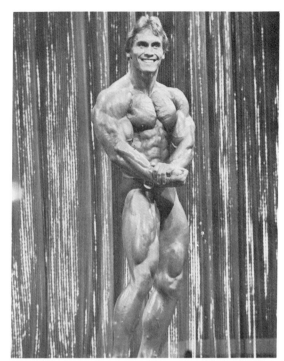

Illus. 307.   Lance Dreher's future as a pro bodybuilder is secured.

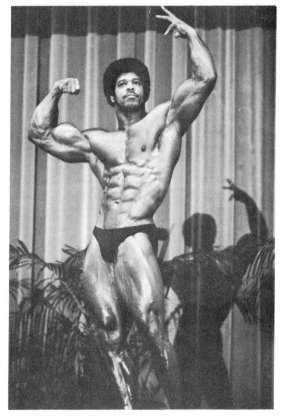

Illus. 308.   Bill Grant's disco routine makes him popular with audiences all over the world.

do justice to your workouts. Sunbathe regularly, but don't overdo it. And don't forget to use sunscreen to protect against burning rays and wrinkles.

I made the mistake of trying steroids last year and really got into them. My strength and development increased rapidly, but I have recently learned from my doctor (who put me on steroids in the first place) that I will have to take thyroid medication for the rest of my life. Why?

Hormones from the thyroid gland are absolutely essential regulating the speed of all your body's internal activities. But if something permanently damages the thyroid gland (as artificial steroids appear to have done in your case), it may stop producing hormones. Then those thyroid hormones must be taken as medication, perhaps as long as you live.

I'm at a point where I've stopped gaining inches and weight. I'm going on 32, am 6'1", 190 pounds. I only started lifting weights in January 1980 and have gained 25 pounds and approximately 24 inches all over my body and have even lost an inch and a half in my waist. I have tried many systems: 1 set of 10 reps, 1 set of 20 reps, 2 × 10, 3 × 10, 5 × 10, 8 × 10. I do 10 reps on average, more and less on certain body parts. I've used light, medium and heavy weights, with the above sets and reps. I do 3 exercises per muscle group. I drink approximately 180 grams of protein three times a day and eat a lot of fish and chicken. Sweets are nonexistent, but I do "garbage out" occasionally. I also take multivitamins several times a day. My rest periods have varied from 30 seconds to 1 minute. I get a good pump more often than not. My work doesn't make heavy physical demands on me, so I'm not burning weight off. Now, don't say anything about sticking points. I haven't stuck—I've stopped. The last gains I made were six months ago. Not everyone can be an Arnold, and I don't expect to be, but I'd like to see something for my effort. Even if I thought that this was all I was going to gain I still wouldn't stop pumping iron. I have been bitten by the bug and it's in my blood.

Your type of problem is extremely common. You appear to be doing everything right, yet progress has come to a halt. This is normal. No one makes continuous gains.

You have made some excellent early gains. My suggestion is to carry on with good, strong, *progressive* workouts using moderately heavy weights

(hoisting up superheavy weights overworks the joints and tendons). Consider using more and more weight since this is definitely a factor in enlarging muscle size. After three or four months of steady training I suggest you "break out" again and go for extra size. Find a new workout partner or a better training facility and *go* for it. See it in your mind . . . feel it . . . taste it. And then blitz your way to the new goal. When it comes, you may have to slow the tempo slightly, consolidate the gains and once again be content to merely hold onto your size for a while. After a few months you can go for a new plateau all over again.

How fast can muscle grow? I want to develop my body in the fastest possible time. I do not want to wait 15 or 20 years to see major changes. How many pounds of muscle can I expect to gain each month?

The average bodybuilder, if he trains hard and eats well, can expect to gain about one pound of muscle per month. With a special surge in training (change of environment, new enthusiasm, new training partner) some seemingly average bodybuilders manage to gain 12 pounds in a month. It all depends on whether you are a natural gainer, and of course on intensity and frequency of workouts and your eating habits. A bodybuilder who has a positive attitude, who sets personal goals, trains regularly and hard, eats three meals a day, takes a good milk-and-egg protein powder and rests sufficiently between workouts, is going to make far better gains than the fellow who has frequent (and unplanned) workouts, skips breakfast, takes no supplements, plays table tennis before his workouts and goes to the disco afterwards.

Mike Mentzer states that very few people can gain even 10 pounds of muscle a year. Mike also pointed out that once your body has "been there," regaining previous mass is quite easy, certainly much easier than the acquisition of new muscle weight. "There exists," says Mentzer, "a 'tissue memory' that makes growth easier the second time around."

Arnold, of course, was a prime example of this phenomenon. He went from 210 to 228 in just over three months to win Mr. Olympia for the sixth time. The most dramatic example of tissue memory, according to Mentzer, was documented by the exercise physiology department of Fort Collins University, Florida. Casey Viator, who had been the 1971 Mr. America, weighed 166 pounds on May 1st, 1973. (He had been injured in an industrial accident and hadn't trained for a long while). Twenty-eight days later, Casey had gained back his best weight . . . 212 pounds. He had added 46 pounds. The actual gain in pure muscle in that one-month period was an incredible 63 pounds—isotope studies revealed that Viator had lost over 17 pounds of fat during the 28-day period. How did he accomplish this gain? Mentzer says: "Casey trained for thirty minutes three times a week for four weeks!" That comes out to a total of 6 *hours* training to gain back 63 pounds of pure muscle mass.

I am having a hard time building my lower thighs. I eat very well, but have "turnip thighs" (heavy at top and small near knee). I do quite a few squats, but only my hips and upper thighs get heavy.

Turnip thighs are caused by poor squatting habits (i.e., leaning too far forward and coming up with backside first or head between knees). Turnip thighs can also be a result of ingesting too many calories. Reduce your food intake. Really muscular thighs (great definition) can seldom be referred to as turnip-shaped. Even though they may be bigger at the top, they rarely look imbalanced.

I suggest you pre-exhaust your thighs by first doing 3 sets of thigh extensions (12 reps), then alternate a further 5 sets of thigh extensions with 5 sets of back squats (heels on 2½-inch blocks, back flat, head up), 10 reps each set.

Finally, immediately after the leg work, take your bike out and cycle up a few steep hills for 10 minutes. Keep to this program for 12 weeks or so, working your thighs every 3 days.

I am a student and just cannot afford any more than 10 minutes a day to train. What is the best single exercise I can do with my barbell set?

Probably the best single exercise would be the squat, clean and press, but even with only 10 minutes a day to train you should do a variety of exercises. No resting between sets. Try splitting your routine working back, legs and abs one day; shoulders, chest and arms the next. Just keep going, nonstop. Your studies are important, but I feel that even so, you should be able to organize your time to manage at least half an hour each day for your workouts.

I have long, gangly arms and I just can't put much meat on them. My biceps have a little size with pretty good peak, but I have a strong desire to add overall arm size as quickly as possible, especially to the triceps. Any suggestions gratefully appreciated.

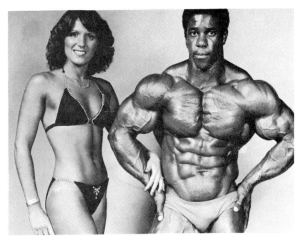

Illus. 309.   Karen Griffiths and Bertil Fox are two of Britain's best.

My present arm workout is seated barbell curls (4 × 12), close-grip concentration curls (4 × 15), standing triceps stretch (4 × 12) and triceps pulley pushdowns (4 × 15).

I feel you are not doing the best arm exercises for size gains. For the next eight weeks I want you to perform only two arm exercises, one for biceps and one for triceps:

1. *Close-Grip Underhand Chin* (5 × 5)

Start each rep with arms totally straight. Don't permit body swing or allow your legs to assist in the chinning. When you can do more than 5 reps, add weight with a dumb-bell between the legs or with the use of a weight belt.

2. *Close-Grip Supine Power Pushes* (5 × 5)

Lying in the bench press position, hold a loaded barbell with a shoulder-width grip. Lower the weight to upper abdomen just below the sternum. Power the weight up with the triceps. To put all the attention on the arms, you *must* keep the elbows close to the body. It should not be long before you are using poundages similar to those used in your regular bench pressing.

After eight weeks you may add two new exercises:

3. *35°-Incline Dumb-bell Curl* (4 × 10)

4. *Lying Triceps Stretch* (4 × 10)

After a while you may find it necessary to review your arm program and adopt an entirely new routine.

Is there any truth to the theory that regular swimming and other mild sports like table tennis or horseback riding will interfere with my bodybuilding gains? I am 5'11" and have worked for seven

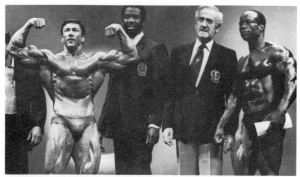

Illus. 310.   Boyer Coe, in winning shape, poses with IFBB secretary Winston Roberts and chairman Ben Weider.

years and only now have 16-inch arms; I'm aiming for 19-inch arms.

You will lose muscle size if you swim and go in for other sports regularly. I say this because your gains have taken quite a long time. An easy gainer, for example, would have gotten 16-inch arms within a couple of years and by five years, 19 inches or so. This means you have to fight like hell to keep your capillaries and muscle cells at their fullest. Extra nonprogressive sports activities will hold back your gains. But if you are blessed with a huge amount of muscle cells and gains come easily, then a moderate amount of extra activity will not hold back gains.

However, even the easy gainer must forget about other sports if he wants to win modern bodybuilding contests. The trick is to get as much muscle size as possible from progressive weight training only, not additional sports. After you become Mr. Universe, you can go in for all the sporting activities you want. Between important contests, you will find Arnold (for example) skiing, playing soccer, skin diving and playing tennis. When he's training to increase muscle size he keeps solely to his workouts.

Is there any way I can prevent getting calluses on my hands from regular bodybuilding with weights?

You could wear gloves. A few bodybuilders (Serge Nubret is one) train with light leather gloves which can be purchased at sporting goods stores. Special weightlifting gloves are not currently available at retail outlets so you should ask for golfer's or race-driving gloves.

I am only 16 and not crazy about building 20-inch arms, but I would always like to be well built and live to a ripe old age. I am greatly in awe of Jack La Lanne. Please tell me how old he is and how he keeps so fit and healthy?

Jack La Lanne is a former hardcore bodybuilder who at 66 now specializes in high energy feats and total fitness. His muscles measure less than they did in his prime, but he still looks very muscular. He will, barring accidents, probably live to the 100 mark. Jack's main recipe for health and fitness is regular weight training combined with swimming or other stamina-building pursuits. Cycling, jogging, rowing, rope-jumping or circuit training (going from one exercise to another, mainly exercising the heart and lungs) are other stamina builders that one could practice. He also believes people in the Western world are living largely on junk foods. "Too many kids are living on soft drinks, sugared desserts and a thousand and one junk foods with chemicals in them." On Jack's list of desirable foods are eggs, fresh fruit, wholewheat bread, salads, raw vegetables (cucumbers, alfalfa sprouts, garbanzo beans, radishes, carrots, mushrooms, onions) baked potatoes (eat the skin too), brown rice, broiled fish, chicken and other poultry. Foods not to be eaten according to Jack include: red meats, pork, fried foods, caffeine (have herbal tea instead), white flour, white and brown sugar, ice cream, sugar-laden candies and cookies. Fitness king Jack also warns us to stay away from pilltaking (aspirin, sleeping pills) when possible. "No tobacco or alcohol at all, and above all keep a positive, vibrant attitude towards life."

Now that the IFBB has declared that a tattoo will subject a competitor to loss of points in competition, please tell me how I can get mine off. I regretted having it put on the day after I got it.

Like a diamond, a professional tattoo is forever. Many plastic surgeons say that there is almost no way to get rid of it without leaving a nasty scar or skin discoloration.

It all depends on how deep into the skin pigment the tattoo is. A 15-minute job by a fly-by-night carnival tattooist will be easier to remove than a real deep pro job. Dermabrasion (sanding) whereby the skin is levelled off layer by layer until the pigment vanishes is the usual treatment, although very small tattoos can be cut out (excised) and the loose skin closed up over it.

I am totally confused. Steve Michalik, Serge Nubret, and even Arnold Schwarzenegger say that you will not build huge muscles using heavy weights, yet men like Mentzer, Scott and Szkalak insist that handling progressively heavier weights will give you the utmost size. Who is right?

Opinions will always vary, but one thing's certain. You can waste years of your bodybuilding life if you don't increase poundages; you have to push the weights at least to a certain stage. Nubret and Arnold both reached 500-pound bench presses. I can also recall seeing Arnold dead-lift 600 and cheat-curl near 300. Michalik has power to spare also.

Every top bodybuilder alive can manage a 300 bench and considerably more on the squat. You simply have to push for more weight during your earlier years in the sport. Later you can moderate the weight used and learn to make the body "feel" the weight even if it is not that heavy.

Try to make your workouts progressive from week to week, year to year. This does not always mean increasing poundage. You can do it by increasing sets, decreasing rest periods, improving style, concentrating on the action, adding reps, tensing and squeezing the muscles at the conclusion of each rep and by adding resistance to the bar, i.e., more weight.

My forearms are so bad I am ashamed to wear a short sleeve shirt. I have developed a pretty good chest and even my upper arms are fair (16¼"), but my forearms are long and skinny with virtually no development.

Many people have difficulty building forearms (and calves) because of insufficient cell allocation in the area. On the other hand, there are thick-wristed "naturals" like Casey Viator, Tim Belknap, Ron Teufel and the Mentzer brothers who never need to do specific forearm work because their forearms grow from regular exercises such as chins, rowing, curls and pulley machines, all of which stimulate and work the forearms strongly.

People such as yourself with "Indian Club" forearms typified by a long wrist appearance and only a small amount of development near the crook of the elbow should work their forearms regularly using the pre-exhaust system.

I suggest you alternate wrist curls, palms down with overgrip chins with hands 6 inches apart, no rest between sets, 4 sets each. Rest briefly and then alternate palms-up wrist curls with undergrip chins, 4 sets of each, no rest between sets.

I do a great number of barbell and dumb-bell presses, but just cannot widen my shoulders. I also do laterals for the lateral (side) head to try to build more width. After every upper body workout my pecs are real sore, but never my delts. And it's delts that I need, especially the side delts.

Start your workouts with 4 quality sets of press-behind-neck-form racks. The exercise builds the entire shoulder area, all 3 heads. Adopt a grip where the lower arms are vertical when bar is raised parallel to the floor. Use a thumbless grip. Keep elbows back. Warm up the shoulder completely, then do 4 heavy (quality) sets of 7 reps. No leanbacks, bouncing or cheating. Next, pre-exhaust by alternating 4 sets of dumb-bell lateral raises with 4 sets of shoulder-width upright rows, 12 reps each set.

When doing the lateral raise, you must perform it either by bending the arms to a right angle (90°), keeping elbows as far back as possible, palms facing the floor throughout the movement, using fairly heavy dumb-bells, or by using relatively light dumb-bells with elbows only slightly bent (unlocked), raising the dumb-bells from a touching together position in front of the body to the arm-raised (slightly above parallel) position. You must keep your hands twisted (little finger uppermost) throughout the movement, and constantly attempt to keep your arms back during the exercise. You will not be able to lift the arms high and this movement will seem extremely awkward, but it works.

The upright rows must also be performed in a specific way to maximize results. Grab the bar with a shoulder-width grip, and as you raise and lower weight, hold it away from the torso, rather than dragging it up touching the body.

I have heard that exercise can cure cancer. Is this true?

No! Exercise cannot cure cancer. But new findings indicate that regular, vigorous exercise can drastically reduce your risk of getting cancer, according to a German study.

Dr. Ernst Van Aaken, author of numerous medical publications, says that his study shows that people who do not exercise are nearly ten times more likely to get cancer than those who exercise strenuously. "Lack of oxygen is one of the key causes of cancer. People who don't exercise run the risk of their healthy cells turning into cancerous tissue." Another test on mice given cancer-promoting chemicals by Dr. Dennis Colacino (University of Wisconsin) showed that the mice given daily exercise on a treadmill developed only half the number of tumors of mice in the sedentary group.

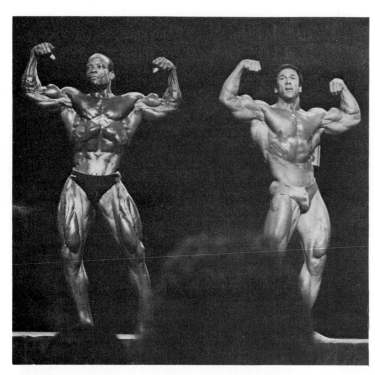

Illus. 311 (left). Al Beckles and Boyer Coe both diet very strictly before a contest to maximize their definition.

Illus. 312 (lower left). Claudia Wilbourn shows a high degree of muscularity.

Illus. 313 (lower right). Strength and muscle blend as one in this picture of Kalman Szkalak.

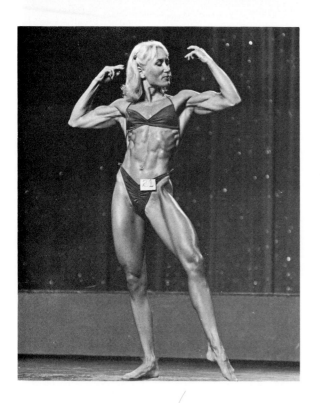

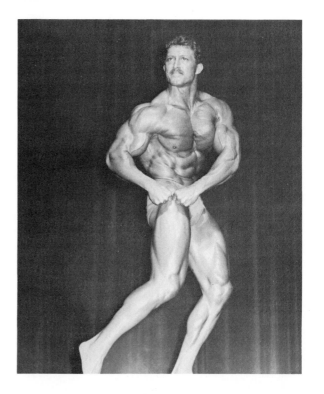

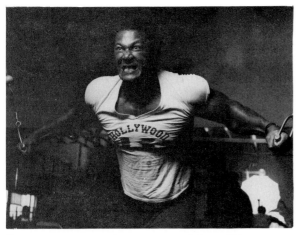

Illus. 314.   Mr. America contestant Manuel Perry performing crossovers.

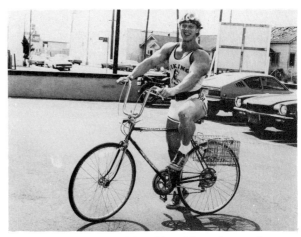

Illus. 315.   Andreas Cahling likes bike riding and combines it with his training when a contest date is coming up.

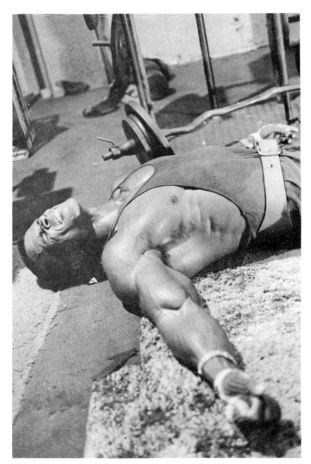

Illus. 316.   Serge Nubret takes a breather after a heavy set of curls.

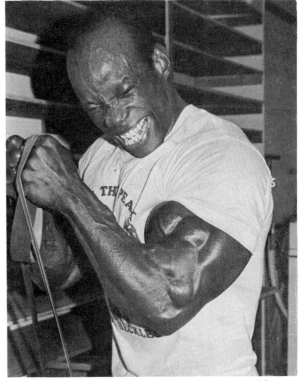

Illus. 317.   Al Beckles carries his own elastic cable, just for pumping, all over the world. That gigantic arm is bringing him worldwide recognition.

Index

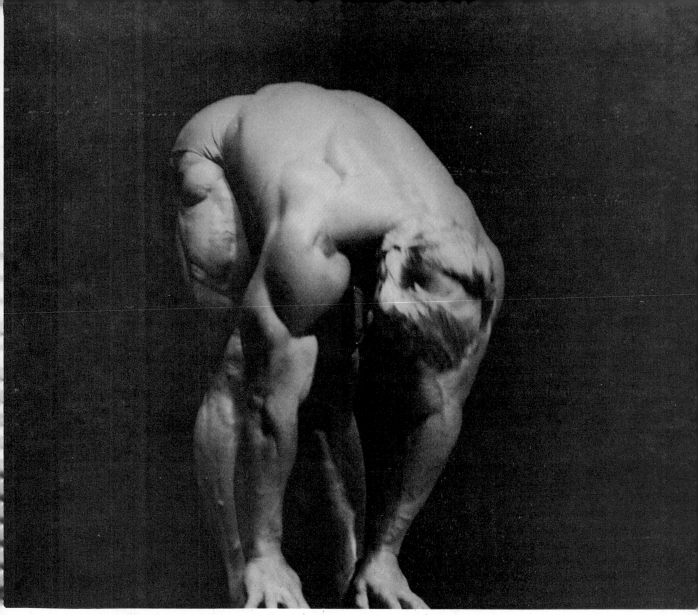

Illus. 318.   The epitome of bodybuilding—Tom Platz.